Stephen L. Isaacs and
David C. Colby, Editors

Foreword by Risa Lavizzo-Mourey

—ᴠᴠ—To Improve Health and Health Care

Volume XIV

The Robert Wood Johnson
Foundation Anthology

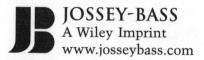

JOSSEY-BASS
A Wiley Imprint
www.josseybass.com

Published by Jossey-Bass
A Wiley Imprint
989 Market Street, San Francisco, CA 94103-1741—www.josseybass.com

Readers should be aware that Internet Web sites offered as citations and/or sources for further information may have changed or disappeared between the time this was written and when it is read.

Jossey-Bass books and products are available through most bookstores. To contact Jossey-Bass directly call our Customer Care Department within the U.S. at 800-956-7739, outside the U.S. at 317-572-3986, or fax 317-572-4002.

Jossey-Bass also publishes its books in a variety of electronic formats. Some content that appears in print may not be available in electronic books.

ISSN: 1547-3570
ISBN 10: 0-4709-2228-1
ISBN 13: 978-04709-2228-6

Printed in the United States of America
FIRST EDITION
PB Printing 10 9 8 7 6 5 4 3 2 1

—⋙—Contents

—✖—Foreword

Risa Lavizzo-Mourey

Each of the past two volumes of *To Improve Health and Health Care: The Robert Wood Johnson Foundation Anthology* has devoted several articles to a single topic. In 2009, the *Anthology* looked at the Foundation's work to promote health insurance for all Americans—a prescient choice given the subsequent enactment of health reform. Last year, it explored lessons that could be learned from programs that did not work out as expected. This year, we turn our attention to a subject that has deep roots in the Robert Wood Johnson Foundation's history and culture: improving the health and health care of vulnerable populations.

The Vulnerable Populations portfolio was created in 2003 as part of a reorganization that took place shortly after we announced a new impact framework designed to make our work more strategic. At the time, we had many programs that focused on the needs of vulnerable populations in their communities and harkened back to the very early days of the Foundation. These programs didn't have a single home. By putting programs in one portfolio, I felt we could do a better job of identifying the best among them.

The Vulnerable Populations portfolio has since created a niche by identifying and supporting innovative programs at the intersection of health and the social factors that influence health—factors such as education, housing, race, class, and income. The portfolio has, for example, supported and helped spread programs to end chronic homelessness,[1] to reduce violence among intimate partners, and to coordinate social services for young people in the juvenile justice system.[2] In this volume, we explore programs to provide mental health services to refugees and immigrants, many of them suffering from posttraumatic stress disorder (see Chapter 4); to curb inner-city gang violence (see Chapter 5); and to bring dental care to Alaskans living in remote areas (see Chapter 6).

More than just supporting these programs, we nurture the most promising among them with the hope and expectation that they can become strong enough to, as David Colby and Stephen Isaacs state in Chapter 1, "enter the mainstream." This volume highlights two innovative programs in the Vulnerable Populations portfolio that we believe have potential to be taken to scale: Playworks, which works with schools to make recess a healthy and fun part of the school day (see Chapter 3), and Green House®, which offers a model of a smaller, more humane kind of nursing home (see Chapter 2).

The Vulnerable Populations programs highlighted in this volume provide a glimpse into our work to improve the health of the neediest of our residents. Other Vulnerable Populations programs have been featured in earlier *Anthology* chapters, as Colby and Isaacs note in the Introduction to Section Two. Collectively, these chapters offer a more complete picture of the Foundation's efforts to improve the health of the nation's most vulnerable individuals.

The Vulnerable Populations portfolio also provides insights into a distinctive form of grantmaking. On the whole, we see strategic philanthropy—the kind that we have practiced in expanding health insurance coverage, reducing tobacco use, and improving end-of-life care—as the way we can have the greatest impact. This kind of strategic grantmaking is often built on a foundation of solid policy research, and Chapter 7 describes the policy research on which the Foundation's efforts to reduce substance abuse rested. Much of the Foundation's impact, however, comes from our Vulnerable Populations work, where we recognize a program that has the potential to dramatically change how services are delivered and at the same time has the potential to help individuals, families, and communities. We want to see that our resources are helping real people make progress toward better health and are moving us toward a healthier society. As this volume makes clear, it is possible, but not always easy, to do both.

Notes

1. Rog, D. J., and Gutman, M. "The Homeless Families Program: A Summary of Key Findings." *To Improve Health and Health Care, 1997: The Robert Wood Johnson Foundation Anthology.* San Francisco: Jossey-Bass, 1997; Diehl, D. "The Homeless Prenatal Program." *To Improve Health and Health Care, Vol. VII: The Robert Wood Johnson Foundation Anthology.* San Francisco: Jossey-Bass, 2004; Bornemeier, J. "The Robert Wood Johnson Foundation Safety Net Programs." *To Improve Health and Health Care, Vol. IX: The Robert Wood Johnson Foundation Anthology.* San Francisco: Jossey-Bass, 2006.
2. Solovitch, S. "Reclaiming Futures." *To Improve Health and Health Care, Vol. XIII: The Robert Wood Johnson Foundation Anthology.* San Francisco: Jossey-Bass, 2010.

—ᴠᴠᴠ—Acknowledgments

We are greatly indebted to all those who contributed to this volume of *To Improve Health and Health Care: The Robert Wood Johnson Foundation Anthology.* In particular, we want to acknowledge the contributions of Elizabeth Dawson, who has done exemplary work as editorial assistant, researcher, proofreader, coordinator, and administrator; Patrick Crow, who has once again proven himself to be without peer as an editor; and Molly McKaughan, who did her usual fine job in reviewing every chapter for accuracy and consistency with Foundation strategy and execution. All three have been associated with the *Anthology* since its inception.

The *Anthology* would not be possible without the stellar efforts of our panel of outside reviewers—Bill Morrill, Patti Patrizi, and Jon Showstack; our fact checker Carolyn Shea; and our editorial consultant Lauren MacIntyre. We thank, as well, Diane Kaplan, Joel Neimeyer, and Steven Schroeder for their helpful comments on various chapters.

Within the Robert Wood Johnson Foundation, we offer our gratitude to David Morse for his guidance throughout the process; Fred Mann for his thoughtfulness and good judgment; Risa Lavizzo-Mourey for her support and counsel; Rose Littman, Chris Clayton, Deb Malloy, and Tina Hynes for their administrative support; Lydia Ryba and Patti Higgins for checking internal program information; Mimi Turi, Mary Castria, Carol Owle, Carolyn Scholer, and Chris Sowa for their management of contractual and financial matters; Ann Christiano, David Krol, and Jane Lowe for reviewing draft chapters; Hope Woodhead and Sherry DeMarchi for overseeing production and distribution; Hinda Greenberg, Mary Beth Kren, and Barbara Sergeant for providing information on a timely basis; and Penny Bolla and the Web team for quickly getting the book on the Foundation's Web site in an attractive and visible format. We wish to single out the especially important contribution Sarah Pickell made to this volume through her conscientious research and fact finding.

At Health Policy Associates, we thank Jay Franz for her book-keeping and contractual oversight. At Jossey-Bass, we acknowledge the many contributions made by Andy Pasternack and his editorial team, Kelsey McGee and Seth Schwartz.

S.L.I. and D.C.C.

Section One
Spreading Innovations

CHAPTER 1

From Idea to Mainstream: The Robert Wood Johnson Foundation Experience

David C. Colby and Stephen L. Isaacs

In the early 1970s, a time when hearses were used to transport sick or injured people to the nearest hospital and getting hold of someone—anyone—who could help in an emergency was a catch-as-catch-can experience, the Robert Wood Johnson Foundation funded one of its first national programs, the Emergency Medical Services Program. It led to the near-universal use of the 911 phone number. To this day, the program offers a model of a foundation-funded program that took off and entered the American mainstream.

The Emergency Medical Services Program was the first, but not the only, example of an idea tested and disseminated by the Foundation that made it into the mainstream. Some ideas were widely replicated and received government funding, thus assuring their continuation. Others became widely accepted and part of the fabric of American society without benefit of legislation. Among the Foundation-supported ideas that have entered the American mainstream are these:

- *Nurse practitioners* were a newly emerging but still marginal profession until the 1970s. Thanks in part to a series of Foundation-funded programs, nurse practitioners became a widely recognized and prestigious profession.[1]

- *Community-based services for people with HIV/AIDS.* In the 1980s, the Foundation tested, in a number of locations, a community-based program that previously served those with AIDS in San Francisco. It became the model for the federal Ryan White Comprehensive AIDS Resources Emergency Act, a law that provides funding for community services for people with HIV/AIDS.[2]

- *Homeless families.* Similarly, the Foundation-Pew Charitable Trusts' Health Care for the Homeless Program served as the model for the McKinney-Vento Act, which funds supportive services for homeless people.[3]

- *Palliative care.* Thanks in part to the support of the Robert Wood Johnson Foundation and the Open Society Institute, palliative care is now a widely accepted element of hospital care.[4]

- *Tobacco control.* The Foundation's efforts in tobacco control in the 1990s are widely credited with playing a role in the dramatic drop in smoking throughout the nation, particularly among young people.[5]

The federal government has adopted and expanded programs initiated by the Foundation. Congress has appropriated funds for programs giving homebound seniors the power to select their own caretakers (Cash & Counseling),[6] enabling Medicaid and insurance companies to team up to give people better long-term care insurance options (Partnership for Long-Term Care),[7] allowing older people the chance to remain at home rather than go to a nursing home (Program of All-Inclusive Care for the Elderly—PACE),[8] and establishing community anti-drug programs (Fighting Back and CADCA).[9, 10] The U.S. Health Services and Resources Administration provides funds for primary care residencies in general medicine and pediatrics, building on pilot programs funded by the Robert Wood Johnson Foundation. Although the programs mentioned above have not yet entered the mainstream, several appear to be poised to do so.

The Nurse-Family Partnership program, in which public health nurses visit young, low-income, first-time mothers in their homes, is another Foundation-funded initiative that may be ready to enter the mainstream.[11] Starting in 1979, the Foundation provided support for a new approach to improving the health of babies and their mothers. In the thirty-one years since its first grant, the Foundation has given nearly $27 million to build evidence about the effectiveness of this approach and to support its replication. In 2002, the Edna McConnell Clark Foundation (along with other foundation and corporate funders, including the Robert Wood Johnson Foundation) funded a major expansion of the program. The recently enacted health reform law authorized $1.5 billion for states that adopt home-visitation programs, such as the Nurse-Family Partnership, that serve young, low-income mothers.

Other Foundation-funded programs appear to have the potential to enter the mainstream, among them programs to develop small and more humane nursing homes (Green House) and to improve the way schools structure recess (Playworks).

—᠊ᨠᨠ᠊— Diffusing Innovations

Why have some programs or ideas worked their way into the mainstream while others have not? What elements have led to their widespread diffusion and adoption? What more can be done to help move good ideas into the mainstream?

These questions have generated considerable thought and debate. Rural sociologist Everett Rogers developed a theory that ideas spread into the mainstream because they are picked up initially by change agents who influence the rest of society until a critical mass of people finds it is in their best interest to adopt an innovation.[12] Economist Walt Rostow coined the term "take-off point"—the accretion of small advances to the point at which change becomes unstoppable—to explain how developing countries grow into developed ones.[13] Malcolm Gladwell observed that the spread of ideas was akin to the spread of a disease; ideas spread through what he calls mavens, connectors, and social marketers. By taking one step at a time, an innovation affects enough people to reach a tipping point, from which it races through the population.[14]

Although these theories are all relevant, they do not explain how ideas advanced by foundations seeking social change go from small, often pilot, efforts to become widely accepted. As Joel Fleishman, former president of the American branch of the Atlantic Philanthropies, observed, "Those foundations that are truly interested in using their resources in ways that will have the greatest positive impact on the world around them should study the stories of the most successful and effective foundation initiatives."[15] The experience of the Robert Wood Johnson Foundation can provide some of those stories.

Emergency Medical Services

As late as the 1960s, emergency medical care was a hodge-podge of different systems—transportation, emergency care, and hospitals—that did not talk to one another. The idea that people having a medical crisis could call a single phone number, wait a short time for an ambulance to show up, and then be transported to a nearby hospital emergency room had not yet entered the public's consciousness.

That began to change in the 1970s. Cities from Miami to Seattle developed systems to dispatch ambulances in response to calls to a specially designated emergency phone number. Scholars began to estimate the number of deaths due to the lack of an emergency medical system (EMS), and the press picked up on this. AT&T designated 911 as *the* emergency number. Trauma care was becoming recognized, and emergency medicine was developing as a field; emergency rooms began to proliferate. Paramedics, having served in Vietnam, were providing care in ambulances taking patients to the nearest emergency room. President Richard Nixon acknowledged the need to improve EMS in his State of the Union address in 1972.

Perhaps most important, millions of television viewers were tuning in to the television show *Emergency!* which featured the exploits of emergency medical system personnel from the Los Angeles County Fire Department saving lives that would have been lost only a short while earlier. "*Emergency!* was the prairie fire," said Eugene Nagel, a Miami physician who was one of the people behind the creation of the EMS system. "The show lit the spark of public awareness."

A new foundation created in 1972—the Robert Wood Johnson Foundation—fanned the flames by working with government and helping to shape development of this new field. Earlier in 1972, the Department of Health, Education, and Welfare had funded EMS demonstration projects at five sites. The Foundation upped the ante by launching the Emergency Medical Services Program to test the EMS concept in forty-four sites and by commissioning the National Academy of Sciences and the RAND Corporation to evaluate it. To run the program, the Foundation named as vice president one of the nation's leading experts in emergency care, Blair Sadler, from the Yale Trauma Program. The Foundation also recruited a high-powered national advisory committee for the program.

At the time, it was possible for a foundation's staff members and executives of the federal government to work hand in glove.

That was exactly what happened. When Congress passed the Emergency Medical Services Systems Act in November 1973, eleven of the fifteen federal components of regional EMS were the same as the components of the Foundation's program. President Gerald Ford appointed David Boyd, a member of the Robert Wood Johnson Foundation's national EMS advisory panel, to run the new Division of Emergency Medical Services at the Department of Health, Education, and Welfare. Emergency medical services experts who were advising the Foundation also advised the federal government. They became advocates for development of a nationwide EMS program—testifying before Congress, writing journal articles, and making radio and television appearances.

Taking advantage of the changing circumstances in the country, the Foundation was instrumental in bringing about change. It built on on steps taken by others, on the public's interest (due largely to the TV show *Emergency!*), and on close collaboration with the federal government. It supported demonstration projects to test EMS in different places, rigorously evaluated the projects, and publicized the results widely. As writer Digby Diehl noted, "In 1976, just 17 percent of the population of the United States had 911 service; by 1979, more than a quarter of the population was served by 911. Today, more than 85 percent of the country is covered by some type of 911 system."[16]

Nurse Practitioners

One of the earliest priorities of the new Robert Wood Johnson Foundation in the early 1970s was to increase the access of people living in rural areas and inner cities to non-hospital care. To advance this priority, the Foundation funded a series of programs to train nurse practitioners and, initially, physician assistants.[17] As early as 1973, the Foundation funded an expansion of a nurse practitioner program at the University of California, Davis that placed emphasis on rural health care. By 1977, more than 230 family nurse practitioners had graduated from that program. That program was followed by the funding of four additional nurse practitioner training programs, with the hope of improving access in underserved areas. The Foundation then made grants to six universities to develop master's degree programs in primary care for nurses; these grants helped the recipients build and sustain the field.

Between 1976 and 1981, the Foundation made small grants to the University of New Mexico to establish guidelines for the training of nurse practitioners. These grants created the basis for accreditation of the new nurse practitioner programs. From 1978 to 1983, the Foundation supplemented this support by funding the training of ninety-nine nurses to be the academic leaders for this new profession. From 1994 to 2004, the Foundation funded the Partnership for Training program with eight sites that used Web and video conferencing to educate 1,140 nurse practitioner, certified nurse midwife, and physician assistant students in underserved areas.

The Foundation's early nurse practitioner efforts were in the forefront of a movement that led to the widespread acceptance of nurse practitioners as recognized health professionals. In many ways, the Foundation's approach to nurse practitioners exemplifies the "disruptive innovations" approach to change articulated by Harvard Business School professor Clayton Christensen.[18] The Foundation supported a less costly group of health professionals, nurse practitioners, who could carry out many of the functions performed by a more costly, and often inaccessible group, namely physicians. A similar disruptive solution to improve access to dental services in Alaska is described in Chapter 6.

AIDS Health Services Program

In 1981, the Centers for Disease Control reported cases of opportunistic diseases among gay men, which we now know to have been acquired immune deficiency syndrome (AIDS). The time between identification of this disease with those first five cases and recognition that one million Americans might have been infected seemed unexpectedly short. Even more disturbing than the numbers was the recognition that there would be no quick cure, treatment, or vaccine for HIV/AIDS.

With no cure in sight, San Francisco developed a community-based model of care for patients with AIDS in the early 1980s. The San Francisco model included a case management system to coordinate care, an AIDS clinic staffed with the necessary professionals, and a community-based counseling and supportive services team staffed by volunteers. The model was expected to provide humane care and prevention education at a reduced cost. Nevertheless, there was concern it could not be replicated in other cities.

In 1986, the Foundation authorized a five-year $17 million grant to test the San Francisco model in eleven other cities. It also funded a rigorous evaluation of the AIDS Health Services Program. Shortly after the Foundation board had authorized the AIDS Health Services Program, the Department of Health and Human Services, responding to a nonbinding "sense of the Congress" resolution highlighting the need for the federal government to do more to address the AIDS crisis, sought the counsel of Robert Wood Johnson Foundation staff members. It developed a four-city AIDS demonstration project (later expanded to twenty-four cities) patterned after the Foundation's program. "The work that the Robert Wood Johnson Foundation was doing," said Sheila McCarthy, a high-ranking official with the U.S. Health Resources and Services Administration (HRSA), "helped HRSA grantees shorten the learning curve and use their funds more efficiently."[19]

In 1990, Congress used the Foundation's AIDS Health Services Program as the model for Title I of the Ryan White Comprehensive AIDS Resources Emergency Act. In their evaluation of the AIDS Health Services Program, Brown University professor Vincent Mor and his colleagues concluded that the program had "shaped public policy by providing examples of certain types of community-based service delivery systems and by creating a climate that favored community-based care."[20]

Tobacco Control

The Surgeon General's report on smoking in 1964, which brought together the research on smoking and health, concluded that cigarettes caused cancer. The report was widely publicized and made a powerful impact throughout the nation. It was followed by other reports by the Surgeon General, most notably one in 1986 that detailed the health hazards of secondhand smoke. With the scientific evidence becoming incontrovertible, the federal government stepped in, requiring that cigarette packs carry warning labels, banning radio and TV ads, and prohibiting smoking on planes. People whose health had been ruined by smoking began to bring lawsuits against tobacco companies. Despite the soothing voices of the tobacco industry, even people who smoked were aware of the risks they were running. From the 1960s on, smoking rates began to decline among adults.

This was the environment in 1991 when the Robert Wood Johnson Foundation made reducing smoking by young people (and implicitly the entire population) one of its priorities. Between 1991 and 2009, the Foundation invested nearly $700 million in its tobacco-control work. Having absorbed some of the lessons from its grantmaking in the 1970s and 1980s, the Foundation adopted a wide-ranging approach. It funded policy research which found that raising taxes on tobacco products resulted in young people buying fewer packs of cigarettes and that banning smoking in public places reduced smoking. In collaboration with the American Medical Association, it developed statewide tobacco-control advocacy coalitions. By requiring matching funds as a condition of these grants, the state coalitions were able to use other, non-Foundation funds to support increases in tobacco taxes, laws banning indoor smoking, and inclusion of cessation treatments in state Medicaid programs and state employee health insurance. The Foundation and its tobacco-control partners also established the Center for Tobacco-Free Kids, a national communications and advocacy organization founded to counter the influence of the powerful Tobacco Institute.

How significant was the Foundation's role in moving tobacco control into the mainstream? Joel Fleishman, author of *The Foundation: A Great American Secret,* listed the Foundation's tobacco control work as one of the twelve highest impact foundation-funded activities of the twentieth century.[21] In a retrospective look at the Foundation's investments in tobacco control, George Grob, president of the Center for Public Program Evaluation, concluded, "Recalling again that any success in the story belongs not only to the Robert Wood Johnson Foundation but also to many collaborators, the results are impressive."[22] The results depended largely on changes in public policy. In seeking to affect policy change, the Foundation employed the full range of tools available to it: policy research and analysis, advocacy, coalition building, convening, and communications, among others.

End-of-Life Care

During the 1970s and 1980s, concern mounted about the care people were receiving toward the end of their lives, especially hospitalized patients being kept alive by machines neither they nor their families wanted. The Right-to-Die Movement and Death with Dignity gained popularity. Dr. Jack Kevorkian took matters one step further by helping people to end their lives. The first hospice in the United States opened in 1974, and Medicare began paying for hospice care in 1982. Words such as *living will* and *health care proxy* entered the language. Two widely publicized court cases—Karen Ann Quinlan, decided by the New Jersey Supreme Court in 1976, and Nancy Cruzan, decided by the United States Supreme Court in 1983—held that a person's desires about medical treatment must be honored, even if it meant ending life support for patients with little or no hope of recovery.

With the great attention being given to end-of-life care, the Robert Wood Johnson Foundation hosted a meeting of experts in 1985 to provide guidance about what contribution the Foundation could make. Out of that meeting grew a large research study called SUPPORT (Study to Understand Prognoses and Preferences for Outcomes and Risks of Treatment) that gave special training to hospital nurses, who would then discuss with terminally ill patients and their families the patient's wishes for care and relay them to physicians. Although the study unearthed a trove of data, the intervention failed. "The problem was not just that physicians were not asking patients their views," wrote Joanne Lynn, the co-principal investigator of SUPPORT. "No one involved talks much—not physicians, families, or patients."[23]

In 1994, SUPPORT's lack of success led the Foundation to embark on a renewed effort to improve the care of seriously ill people. The Foundation, in an informal collaboration with the Open Society Institute, employed a full range of strategies to improve end-of-life care. It worked to add end-of-life care to medical and nursing licensing examinations and to incorporate material on end-of-life care in medical and nursing textbooks and curricula. It funded fellowships in palliative medicine and promoted hospital-based palliative care, mainly through the Center to Advance Palliative Care located at the Mount Sinai School of Medicine in New York City, which became a national resource center. The Foundation funded efforts to rally advocates and to support coalitions of concerned individuals, and it developed an active communications program, the centerpiece of which was a widely watched PBS special hosted by Bill Moyers called *On Our Own Terms*.

By 2010, palliative care had become part of mainstream medical care, an option available to very sick hospital patients and their families. Three-quarters of hospitals with 250 or more beds (that is, hospitals serving the majority of America's patients) reported having a palliative care program, and 30 percent of all hospitals had one. In 2006, the American Board of Medical Specialties recognized palliative medicine as a medical subspecialty. In a review of the Foundation's work on end-of-life care, Patricia Patrizi and her colleagues concluded, "The Foundation's impact transcended any possible list of discrete accomplishments. In fact, most credit the Foundation with 'building the field' of end-of-life care."[24]

—ᴧᴧ— Four Elements Needed to Move Foundation-Funded Ideas into the Mainstream

The experience of the Robert Wood Johnson Foundation indicates that four elements are usually present when an idea takes hold and makes it into the mainstream. This does not mean that an idea will necessarily take hold when all four of these elements are present, nor does it mean that an idea will not be widely adopted in the absence of one or more of these. But it does offer a perspective, based on the experience of one foundation, on how ideas get widely diffused and on what philanthropy can do to spur the process. The key ingredients are as follows.

1. *The idea is seen by a substantial portion—or at least an influential portion—of the population as a potential solution to a pressing problem.*

Lack of emergency medical care, an AIDS epidemic, people dying from tobacco use or exposure, shortages of health professionals, individuals in hospitals tethered to machines that preserve life but do not restore the quality of life—these issues had entered Americans' consciousness, in some cases had generated movements, and were ripe for action to address them. As it happened, methods of alleviating these problems were widely recognized, and they were tested in a variety of locations. The emergency medical system benefited from both government-funded and Foundation-funded demonstration projects. The lack of medical services in rural areas and inner cities was addressed, in part at least, by employing nurse practitioners who would actually spend some time in these areas. Although there was no cure for AIDS, San Francisco offered a model for caring for those who were HIV-positive. In testing that model, the Foundation showed it could work in places with different health systems and cultures. By the 1990s, the health hazards of smoking were widely known, and actions to help people quit (or not start) were obvious and ready for adoption on a wide scale.

In all of these cases, the Robert Wood Johnson Foundation understood the importance of the issues to Americans, seized the initiative, and helped direct and shape the strategies to address the issues.

2. The political system is receptive to the adoption of new ideas—especially when legislation is the means of spreading them.

Ideas that took hold in the 1970s, such as emergency medical services and nurse practitioners, were products of a period when government could be expected to adopt worthy demonstration programs and expand them nationwide. During this time, government and foundations collaborated on a regular basis and experts moved between senior government positions and national advisory committees of foundation-funded programs. In that context, it is not surprising the federal government would assume responsibility for adopting innovative programs such as EMS and funding the education of primary care providers, including nurse practitioners.

Even when political leaders see the government as the problem rather than as a promoter of solutions, however, it is still possible to spread innovations with government help and guidance. The Ryan White Act was adopted in part because of the intense pressure on Congress generated by the AIDS crisis and because Congress responded on a bipartisan basis. The Cash & Counseling program, which, because it allowed frail elders and adults with disabilities to choose the way to meet their personal care needs under Medicaid, was attractive to a Republican President and Congress and was authorized in the Deficit Reduction Act of 2005. The same is true of the Partnership for Long-Term Care, which was also adopted as part of the 2005 Deficit Reduction Act.

3. *The evidence is strong that an idea is workable and perhaps cost-effective.*

In all of the cases we have discussed, evidence of an idea's feasibility was strong and, in some cases, overwhelming. Nurse practitioners, for example, were shown to deliver primary care comparable to that of physicians and at a far lower cost; AIDS services could be delivered effectively and relatively cheaply in the community; tobacco taxes reduced smoking and saved lives; Cash & Counseling gave homebound seniors control of their care and reduced Medicaid costs for participants; and palliative care was shown to be cost-effective care. These social policy changes were all built on a strong evidence base.

Unlike the political-economic environment and public opinion, over which foundations have little direct influence, foundations can develop and strengthen the evidence base, which, if disseminated properly, can sway opinions and environments. The Substance Abuse Policy Research Program discussed in Chapter 7 provides an excellent illustration of how a strong research base can influence policy. Similarly, random-controlled trials in Elmira, Memphis, and Denver demonstrating the cost-effectiveness of the Nurse-Family Partnership program led to its expansion. Solid evidence based on research does not, of course, ensure action will be taken. But without evidence, action is unlikely.

4. *Committed advocates keep the idea in the forefront and fight for its widespread adoption.*

Advocates and advocacy organizations have often served as the link between the research and policy-making communities. In the case of Foundation-supported ideas that have taken hold, passionate advocates, most outside of government but some inside, have made change possible. William Novelli and Matt Myers at the Center for Tobacco-Free Kids confronted the tobacco companies; Philip Brickner, a physician at St. Vincent's Hospital and Medical Center in New York City, was a tireless advocate for the homeless. His efforts influenced the McKinney-Vento Act; Mervyn Silverman fought to expand the community-based approaches to care for people with AIDS he had instituted as San Francisco commissioner of health.

Advocates are the ones who keep the issue alive, who don't let the public forget, and who fight to turn ideas into law.

—⚓— Identifying and Nurturing the Next Blockbuster Ideas

Just as pharmaceutical companies look for a blockbuster drug, so, too, do foundations look for blockbuster ideas that will, at the very least, be sustained by government funding and, even better, become part of normal American life. But not all ideas have the potential to become widely accepted. Foundations should be rigorous in identifying ideas that have the potential to enter the mainstream and should not waste resources promoting those that are unlikely to make it. A number of promising Robert Wood Johnson Foundation–funded ideas and programs may be poised to become widely replicated and accepted. They include the following:

- *Smaller, more humane nursing homes.* The Green House Program has shown great potential in improving the lives of frail seniors. As Irene Wielawski writes in this volume,[25] the program may be the wave of the future—or it may simply become an adjunct to large, impersonal nursing homes.

- *Better care for pregnant women and newborns.* Consistently evaluated as a cost-effective program to improve the health of children born to impoverished mothers, the nurse-family partnership program was initially funded by the Robert Wood Johnson Foundation and has received significant additional support, including support from the Edna McConnell Clark Foundation and, more recently, from the federal government. The program is currently active in thirty-one states.

- *Better nutrition and more physical activity for children.*
  The Foundation is committed to reversing the
  childhood obesity epidemic and has committed
  $500 million to the effort. Although reversing the
  obesity trend presents a major challenge, many of the
  elements common to widespread adoption of an idea
  are in place; attitudes are already changing, and the
  Foundation's impact could be similar to its impact in
  tobacco control.

- *Greater attention to the benefits of play and recess in
  schools.* The Playworks program that the Foundation
  has supported since 2005 appears to have the potential
  to spread widely. Whether it becomes part of the mainstream may depend, as Carolyn Newbergh observes
  in Chapter 3, on whether school districts see it as a
  priority in difficult economic times.

- *Improved quality and lower-cost medical care.* Concern
  about expanding health insurance coverage drove
  much of the health care reform debate in 2009
  and 2010. Improving quality and lowering cost
  were part—but a lesser part—of that debate. The
  Foundation has a long track record in trying to
  advance high-quality, cost-effective systems of care,
  dating back to its support of the National Committee
  on Quality Assurance and the Dartmouth Atlas.
  With enactment of health reform, the time may be
  approaching when quality will make it to the top of the
  health care agenda. If this happens, the Foundation's
  investments over many years will be something to
  build on.

- *Accrediting public health departments.* The Foundation has been supporting efforts to develop standards
  for public health departments and an organization to
  accredit the departments. Although these efforts are
  not as visible to the public as many other Foundation
  initiatives, they could be instrumental in improving the
  quality of public health departments and the services
  they provide.

Whether these ideas or others become the next blockbusters, there are certain steps foundations can take to nurture ideas and increase their chances of making it into the mainstream, including the following:

1. Identify ideas that have the potential to enter the mainstream and help shape the course of their development.

2. Use all of the tools available to philanthropy. The president and CEO of the Robert Wood Johnson Foundation, Risa Lavizzo-Mourey, has defined these in terms of the "Five C's"—communicating, convening, coordinating, connecting, and counting—plus a sixth, cash.[26]

3. Nurture people. Organizations are important, but it is individual advocates, researchers, policy makers, and other leaders who move ideas. Human capital is important.

4. Support independent research to provide an evidence base that will be widely accepted.

5. Communicate promising ideas widely. For foundations interested in shaping public policy and affecting social change, communications is a key tool.

6. Stick with good ideas for a long time. An inhospitable political climate can suddenly become inviting, as the passage of health care reform in 2010 demonstrates.

Notes

1. Keenan, T. "Support of Nurse Practitioners and Physician Assistants." *To Improve Health and Health Care, 1998–1999: The Robert Wood Johnson Foundation Anthology.* San Francisco: Jossey-Bass, 1998.
2. Bronner, E. "The Foundation and AIDS: Behind the Curve but Leading the Way." *To Improve Health and Health Care, Vol. V: The Robert Wood Johnson Foundation Anthology.* San Francisco: Jossey-Bass, 2002.
3. Bornemeier, J. "The Robert Wood Johnson Foundation's Safety Net Programs." *To Improve Health and Health Care, Vol. IX: The Robert Wood Johnson Foundation Anthology.* San Francisco: Jossey-Bass, 2006.

4. Meier, D. E., Isaacs, S. L., and Hughes, R. G., eds. *Palliative Care: Transforming the Care of Serious Illness.* San Francisco, Jossey-Bass, 2010.

5. Bornemeier, J. "Taking on Tobacco: The Robert Wood Johnson Foundation's Assault on Smoking." *To Improve Health and Health Care, Vol. VIII: The Robert Wood Johnson Foundation Anthology.* San Francisco: Jossey-Bass, 2005.

6. Benjamin, A. E., and Snyder, R. E. "Consumer Choice in Long-Term Care." *To Improve Health and Health Care, Vol. V: The Robert Wood Johnson Foundation Anthology.* San Francisco: Jossey-Bass, 2002.

7. Alper, J. "The Partnership for Long-Term Care: A Public-Private Partnership to Finance Long-Term Care." *To Improve Health and Health Care, Vol. X: The Robert Wood Johnson Foundation Anthology.* San Francisco: Jossey-Bass, 2006.

8. Alper, J., and Gibson, R. "Integrating Acute and Long-Term for the Elderly." *To Improve Health and Health Care, 2001: The Robert Wood Johnson Foundation Anthology.* San Francisco: Jossey-Bass, 2001.

9. Wielawski, I. M. "The Fighting Back Program." *To Improve Health and Health Care, Vol. VII: The Robert Wood Johnson Foundation Anthology.* San Francisco: Jossey-Bass, 2004.

10. Jellinek, P., and Schapiro, R. "Join Together and CADCA: Back up the Front Line." *To Improve Health and Health Care, Vol. VII: The Robert Wood Johnson Foundation Anthology.* San Francisco: Jossey-Bass, 2004.

11. Alper, J. "The Nurse Home Visitation Program." *To Improve Health and Health Care, Vol. V: The Robert Wood Johnson Foundation Anthology.* San Francisco: Jossey-Bass, 2002.

12. Rogers, E. *Diffusion of Innovations* (4th ed.). New York: Free Press, 1995.

13. Rostow, W. W. *The Stages of Economic Growth.* Cambridge: Cambridge University Press, 1960.

14. Gladwell, M. *The Tipping Point: How Little Things Can Make a Big Difference.* New York: Little, Brown, 2000.

15. Fleishman, J. A. *The Foundation: A Great American Secret.* New York: Public Access, 2007, p. 159.

16. Diehl, D. "The Emergency Medical Services Program." *To Improve Health and Health Care, 2000: The Robert Wood Johnson Foundation Anthology.* San Francisco: Jossey Bass, 2000.

17. The Foundation continued supporting nurse practitioners for many years, but it did not continue its support of physician assistants.

18. Christensen, C. *The Innovator's Dilemma.* Cambridge, Mass.: Harvard Business School Press, 1997.

19. Health Resources and Services Administration, U.S. Department of Health and Human Services. "HRSA Funds First AIDS Program at $15.3 Million," 1986. http://hab.hrsa.gov/livinghistory/timeline/1986.htm.

20. Mor, V., Fleishman, J. A., Allen, S. M., and Piette, J. *Networking AIDS Services.* Ann Arbor, MI: Health Administration Press, 1994, p. 214.

21. Fleishman, *The Foundation.*

22. Grob, G. *The Tobacco Campaigns of the Robert Wood Johnson Foundation and Its Collaborators, 1991–2009.* (Report to the Robert Wood Johnson Foundation). Center for Public Program Evaluation, December 2009.

23. Lynn, J. "Unexpected Returns." *To Improve Health and Health Care, 1997: The Robert Wood Johnson Foundation Anthology.* San Francisco: Jossey Bass, 1997.

24. Patrizi, P., Thompson, E., and Spector, A. "Death Is Certain. Strategy Isn't: Assessing RWJF's End-of-Life Grantmaking," presented at the Strategy Forum of the Evaluation Roundtable, May 21–23, 2008, p. 52.

25. See Chapter 2.

26. Lavizzo-Mourey, R. "Foreword." *To Improve Health and Health Care: The Robert Wood Johnson Foundation Anthology, Vol. IX.* San Francisco: Jossey-Bass, 2006.

Section Two
Vulnerable Populations

Editors' Introduction to Section Two

Vulnerable Populations

This section of the *Anthology* features five chapters highlighting programs from the Foundation's Vulnerable Populations portfolio—the part of the Foundation that works at the intersection of health and the social and economic factors that influence it, or, as stated on the Foundation's Web site, that "create new opportunities for better health by investing in health where it starts—in our homes, schools and jobs."[1]

The chapters that follow illustrate the Foundation's commitment to improving the care of seniors (Green House Program); children (Playworks); immigrants and refugees (Caring Across Communities); and people living in remote, underserved areas (Dental Health Aides and Therapists), as well as its efforts to reduce inner-city gang violence (United Teen Equality Center). These represent only a small sample of the kinds of programs supported by the Vulnerable Populations portfolio. Earlier volumes of the *Anthology* series have examined other programs to improve services for or conditions of vulnerable populations, including homeless people,[2] people in trouble with the law,[3] seniors,[4] children and adolescents,[5] needy people living in New Jersey,[6] Native Americans,[7] and people victimized by natural disasters.[8] The exhibit on the following page lists programs to improve the health of vulnerable populations of more than $1 million.

The Foundation's staff members have worked to ensure that some of these creative approaches become part of the mainstream. That involves identifying breakthrough approaches, testing them at pilot sites, and preparing some of them for widespread adoption. As Risa Lavizzo-Mourey observes in her foreword to this volume, the Foundation's Vulnerable Populations portfolio and its predecessors have been a proving ground for developing creative approaches to improve the lives of the nation's neediest people—approaches that have been and can be expanded to reach significant numbers of America's most vulnerable populations.

Vulnerable Populations Program Investments of More Than $1 Million Since 2003

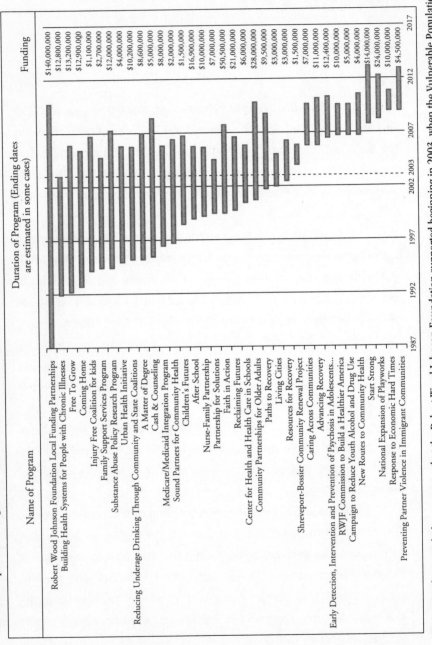

Note: **This figure includes programs that the Robert Wood Johnson Foundation supported beginning in 2003, when the Vulnerable Populations portfolio was established. It indicates the date when the Foundation's support began and is currently scheduled to end.**

Notes

1. The Robert Wood Johnson Foundation. "Vulnerable Populations." 2010. http://www .rwjf.org/vulnerablepopulations/index.jsp.

2. Rog, J. R., and Gutman, M. "The Homeless Families Program: a Summary of Key Findings." *To Improve Health and Health Care, 1997: The Robert Wood Johnson Foundation Anthology*. San Francisco: Jossey-Bass, 1997; Bornemeier, J. "The Robert Wood Johnson Foundation's Safety Net Programs." *To Improve Health and Health Care, Vol. IX: The Robert Wood Johnson Foundation Anthology*. San Francisco: Jossey-Bass, 2006; Diehl, D. "The Homeless Prenatal Program." *To Improve Health and Health Care, Vol. VII: The Robert Wood Johnson Foundation Anthology*. San Francisco: Jossey-Bass, 2004.

3. Bunch, W. "Helping Former Prisoners Reenter Society: The Health Link Project." *To Improve Health and Health Care, Vol. XII: The Robert Wood Johnson Foundation Anthology*. San Francisco: Jossey-Bass, 2009; Solovitch, S. "Reclaiming Futures." *To Improve Health and Health Care, Vol. XIII: The Robert Wood Johnson Foundation Anthology*. San Francisco: Jossey-Bass, 2009.

4. Allen, S. M., and Mor, V. "Unmet Need in the Community: The Springfield Study." *To Improve Health and Health Policy, 1997: The Robert Wood Johnson Foundation Anthology*. San Francisco: Jossey-Bass, 1997; Jellinek, P., Appel, T. G., and Keenan, T. "Faith in Action." *To Improve Health and Health Care, 1998–1999: The Robert Wood Johnson Foundation Anthology*. San Francisco: Jossey-Bass, 1998; Alper, J. "Coming Home: Affordable Assisted Living for the Rural Elderly." *To Improve Health and Health Care, 2000: The Robert Wood Johnson Foundation Anthology*. Jossey-Bass, 1999; Smyth, H. R., Cox, N. J., Reifler, B. V., and Ashbury, C. "Adult Day Centers." *To Improve Health and Health Care, 2000: The Robert Wood Johnson Foundation Anthology*. San Francisco: Jossey-Bass, 1999; Alper, J., and Gibson, R. "Integrating Acute and Long-Term Care for the Elderly." *To Improve Health and Health Care, 2001: The Robert Wood Johnson Foundation Anthology*. San Francisco: Jossey-Bass, 2001; Benjamin, A. E., and Snyder, R. E. "Consumer Choice in Long-Term Care." *To Improve Health and Health Care, Vol. V: The Robert Wood Johnson Foundation Anthology*. San Francisco: Jossey- Bass, 2002; Dentzer, S. "Service Credit Banking." *To Improve Health and Health Care, Vol. V: The Robert Wood Johnson Foundation Anthology*. San Francisco: Jossey-Bass, 2002; Bronner, E. "The Teaching Nursing Home Program." *To Improve Health and Health Care, Vol. VII: The Robert Wood Johnson Foundation Anthology*. San Francisco: Jossey-Bass, 2004; Mockenhaupt, R. E., Lower, J. I., and Magan, G. G. "Improving Health in an Aging Society." *To Improve Health and Health Care, Vol. IX: The Robert Wood Johnson Foundation Anthology*. San Francisco: Jossey-Bass, 2006; Alper, J. "The Partnership for Long-Term Care: A Public-Private Partnership to Finance Long-Term Care." *To Improve Health and Health Policy: The Robert Wood Johnson Foundation Anthology, Vol. IX*. San Francisco: Jossey-Bass, 2006.

5. Begley, S., and Hearn, R. P. "Children's Health Initiative." *To Improve Health and Health Care, 2001: The Robert Wood Johnson Foundation Anthology.* San Francisco: Jossey-Bass, 2001; Brodeur, P. "Students Run LA." *To Improve Health and Health Care, Vol. IX: The Robert Wood Johnson Foundation.* San Francisco: Jossey-Bass, 2006; Wielawski, I. M. "Mentoring Young People." *To Improve Health and Health Policy, Vol. XI: The Robert Wood Johnson Foundation Anthology.* San Francisco: Jossey-Bass, 2008.

6. Dickson, P. S. "Tending Our Backyard: The Robert Wood Johnson Foundation's Grantmaking in New Jersey." *To Improve Health and Health Care, Vol. V: The Robert Wood Johnson Foundation Anthology.* San Francisco: Jossey-Bass, 2002.

7. Brodeur, P. "Programs to Improve the Health of Native Americans." *To Improve Health and Health Care, Vol. V: The Robert Wood Johnson Foundation Anthology.* San Francisco: Jossey-Bass, 2002; Brodeur, P. "Fighting Back and Healthy Nations in Gallup, New Mexico." *To Improve Health and Health Care, Vol. VI: The Robert Wood Johnson Foundation Anthology.* San Francisco: Jossey-Bass, 2006.

8. Isaacs, S. L. and Rogers, J. H. "Partnership Among National Foundations: Between Rhetoric and Reality." *To Improve Health and Health Care, 2001: The Robert Wood Johnson Foundation Anthology.* San Francisco: Jossey-Bass, 2001.

CHAPTER 2

The Green House® Program

Irene M. Wielawski

Editors' Introduction

How does one care for older people in a society that does not respect or value age? Finding the answer to this question presents a major challenge, one that will only grow more difficult as the population ages. Already, 10 million Americans receive some form of long-term care assistance, and as many as 44 million relatives and friends are helping them. The cost is staggering, both in personal and financial terms: long-term care consumes more than $200 billion a year in government spending—and this doesn't count the hundreds of billions of dollars families contribute in time and money.

An overwhelming percentage of seniors prefer to remain at home or live in their communities. This explains the great interest in home-health care (now the fastest rising part of the Medicaid budget) and community-based care, such as adult day centers, congregate living facilities, and continuing care retirement communities.

Nursing homes are widely considered to be a last resort; they are often thought of as large, cold institutions where old people go to die. This stereotype is true to a great extent, but some aspects of nursing home care are changing. One of the changes is represented by Green House, a smaller and kinder sort of nursing home. Green House is the brainchild of a visionary geriatrician named Bill Thomas, who originally developed the concept with the support of the Fan Fox and Leslie R. Samuels Foundation. In 2002, the Robert Wood Johnson Foundation awarded $305,000 to Thomas's organization to advocate for and test the Green House idea in Utica, New York. That test didn't happen, as this chapter explains, but the seed was planted. Steve McAllily, head of the United Methodist Senior Services of Mississippi, heard Thomas speak, experienced his own conversion, and decided to replace United Methodist's Cedars nursing home in Tupelo, Mississippi, with twelve Green Houses. The Green Houses were opened in Tupelo, Mississippi, in 2003. Since that time, the Foundation has awarded nearly $12 million, primarily to NCB Capital Impact, to develop, test, and evaluate the concept, which has received wide praise as an innovative approach to caring for the frail elderly.

In this chapter, Irene Wielawski, a veteran investigative reporter and a founder of the Association of Health Care Journalists, examines the Green House Program. She explores the beginnings and development of the idea, reports on visits to two Green Houses, and concludes by offering some thoughts on the viability of Green Houses as an alternative to traditional nursing homes.

—ɯ— **S**tanley Radzyminski remembers the Army fondly, but not for the three years he served in the China-Burma-India Theater during World War II. Rather, it's for the day he reported for duty as a stenotype operator and caught the attention of the officer in charge. Like Radzyminski, the officer was from a large Polish-American family, and in a subsequent letter home suggested that his sister, Edna, write to the "nice Polish boy" in his unit.

The letters were the beginning of a lifelong romance. The couple married in 1947 and, unable to have children, lived in singular devotion to each other. They bought a two-family house in Radzyminski's hometown of Albany, New York and grew old together, secure in the routines of their long, shared life. That is, until the day Radzyminski arrived home to find his wife lying unconscious in a pool of blood.

She had slipped and fallen, fracturing her skull, a shoulder, and both arms. Surgical repairs and six months in a rehabilitation facility enabled her to return home, and the couple, now well into their eighties, were able to manage for a while with the help of visiting nurses. But then Stanley and Edna both fell as they tried to unfold her wheelchair, and neither could get up. Rescue crews took them to the hospital, and from there they joined the ranks of some 1.5 million Americans living in nursing homes.[1]

The Radzyminskis' entry into residential care was fairly typical; experts cite injury, debilitating illness, and dementia or other cognitive impairment as the chief reasons for this transition from independent living to institutional care. At one time, the Radzyminskis' accidents might have forced them into separate facilities specializing in their particular medical needs. (Edna developed dementia and had difficulty communicating.) But they remained together until Edna died in 2010, thanks in part to an innovative residential care model called Green House®.

Green Houses, at first glance, seem to be a radical departure from the hospital-like fortresses most people associate with nursing homes. They're designed to look like suburban ranch houses. (The cluster of Green Houses in upstate New York where the Radzyminskis live could easily be mistaken for a middle-income housing development.) Each Green House has no more than twelve residents and operates to foster a sense of community among residents and staff, while also de-emphasizing the top-down hierarchy of traditional nursing homes.

Their charismatic founder, the geriatrician William H. Thomas, who calls himself a "nursing home abolitionist," describes Green Houses as the antithesis of the "ageism and declinism" that permeate traditional long-term care institutions. Thomas sees old age, despite the infirmities and disabilities that accompany this stage of life, as simply another phase of human growth and development, which ought to be supported by the environments in which old people live. Skeptics, meanwhile, say Green House is a boutique concept that has yet to prove versatile enough to accommodate the spectrum of old people's health and safety needs at reasonable cost.

In 2002, the Robert Wood Johnson Foundation began a series of grant-funded investigations into the viability of such small community-based nursing homes. By mid-2010, eighty-nine Green Houses were up and running, partly as a result of the Foundation's support. But Green Houses remain very much a work in progress for early adopters, who have been propelled by Thomas's vision into terrain with few scientific markers but many passions. Those passions reflect not only our unease with old age and impending death but also our unease with deficiencies in the status quo.

—⁓— Who Wants to Live in a Nursing Home?

In a 2007 public opinion survey by the Kaiser Family Foundation, only 4 percent of respondents said they would opt for nursing home care. About 75 percent said they would prefer to remain in their homes with assistants or to move in with relatives if they could no longer care for themselves. Even more damning were responses to a question about whether they believed nursing home residents are better or worse off than they were before they left their homes. Only 19 percent thought people benefited from nursing home care, whereas 41 percent said being in the nursing home made people "worse off than they were before."[2]

Pretty low marks for an industry that accounts for more than $130 billion in state and federal expenditures alone.[3] And it's not just lacerating polling data or the latest exposé of terrible conditions that has given nursing homes a bad name. Today's nursing homes have spent nearly a quarter century under an official cloud—ever since an Institute of Medicine (IOM) report in 1986 described a failed system of state and federal oversight and wide variation in the quality of care.[4] The IOM report detailed widespread dissatisfaction with the status quo.

Congress responded with reform legislation, embedded in the Omnibus Budget Reconciliation Act (OBRA) of 1987. The Health Care Financing Administration (now called the Centers for Medicare & Medicaid Services) followed up in the early 1990s with regulations that were focused on residents. Among other things, nursing homes were required to develop individualized care plans with an overall goal of helping residents achieve their best possible physical and mental function.

OBRA 1987 routinely receives star billing when experts talk about improvements in the quality of long-term care. But although improved regulations and better oversight have helped, they're by no means the sole reason for a greatly improved and still transforming industry today. Market factors and an aging long-term care infrastructure combined with a growing *culture change* movement have opened the field to experimental and innovative ideas like Green House.

Perhaps the greatest stimulus (considering that for-profit companies operate most of the nursing homes in the United States) is the graying of the Baby Boom generation. This population bulge—demographers call it "the pig in the python"[5]—has loomed over every long-term care initiative since the first White House Conference on Aging in 1961. Baby Boomers were born between 1946 and 1964,[6] meaning they'll begin to cross the threshold of old age in 2011. Demands on the nation's health and social welfare system are projected to increase steadily, even as there are proportionately fewer workers contributing to these largely tax-financed programs. In raw figures, the number of Americans aged 65 and older is expected to reach 81 million by 2040, double what it is today.[7] About 70 percent of Americans are expected to need some form of long-term care services during their lifetime.[8]

Of more immediate concern is the poor physical condition of many of the nation's 16,100 certified nursing facilities. Most were constructed in the decade following Congress's passage of Medicare and Medicaid in 1965—which included money for rehabilitation and convalescent care—and are due for renovation. This need has opened the door to new ideas in nursing home design and function. The older model was fashioned on hospitals, partly because of the dictates of regulations governing the construction of health care facilities. As a result, even though the idea was to build "homes" for frail or sick people who could no longer live independently, what emerged were big buildings that looked like hospitals. They also ran like hospitals, with semiprivate rooms, rigid schedules for residents' wake-up and bedtimes, meals, exercise, and so on, with many hierarchical layers of supervision and authority.

"Before the building boom in the 1960s and '70s, there were the old-fashioned rest homes for the aged, with overstuffed chairs, private bedrooms, and gang bathrooms," recalls Monsignor Charles J. Fahey, a Catholic priest and scholar at Fordham University who chairs the National Council on Aging. "There were also private homes, often [owned by] a nurse and her husband, who took elderly people in for income."

In scale and ambiance, new concepts like Green House aren't so different from this nineteenth- and early-twentieth-century model. But they're intended to go beyond simply a homey look to create an environment that supports residents' self-determination, dignity, and life goals, while also delivering twenty-first-century medical care. These environmental principles are the hallmark of the culture-change movement in long-term care. The people behind it are a diverse group that includes consumers, nursing home administrators, and medical professionals like Bill Thomas, who are loosely affiliated through an organization called the Pioneer Network, which was founded in 1997. Even an "abolitionist" like Thomas acknowledges the resulting improvements in traditional nursing homes.

"Institutional long-term care facilities are radically better than they were twenty years ago," he says, noting a lag in public recognition, as evidenced by opinion polls like Kaiser's, and also the influence of human psychology on poll results. "The results in every survey of older people are staggering. If you ask them what they are afraid of, death comes in third; the top two are being placed in a nursing home and loss of independence. People abhor and dread the prospect of institutionalization. The vast majority will say, 'I want to live at home,' even if that means living alone without the social opportunities of a well-functioning institution."

Which is why Thomas wants the hospital-like structures replaced by Green Houses.

"There is no other way," he says. "A nursing home is still an institution. There's a deeply flawed view of humanity that occurs in those buildings. To be generous, it's an asylum mentality that prevails in nursing homes, as in prisons or state psychiatric hospitals."

—ᴟ— The Green House Idea Takes Shape

In calling for the abolition of nursing homes and all forms of *institutionalization* of the aged and infirm, Thomas speaks to people's highest aspirations for ailing loved ones as well as to their deepest fears about the setting and conditions of their own demise. He has written several books and has lectured widely on his vision of a more humanistic model of care for the frail elderly. His passion for this idea is described by many as compelling—and infectious.

Laurie Mante, an administrator on the nursing home side of Northeast Health, a not-for-profit health care organization based in Troy, New York, remembers being so mesmerized by one of Thomas's speeches that she returned to her job determined to demolish the facility that employed her—which she has largely succeeded in doing.

"I'm a fidget, can't sit still and just listen, so my usual thing at lectures is to plunk down on a chair in the back and go through my mail," Mante recalls. "All I can tell you is once Bill Thomas started talking, I never opened a single envelope."

Thomas similarly captivated the Robert Wood Johnson Foundation. Longtime program officers still recall his first visit in 2001 to their staid Princeton, New Jersey, headquarters, where deferential grant applicants typically show up in business suits. Thomas, whose home is a working farm in upstate New York, wore jeans, a sweatshirt, and Birkenstock sandals. Recalling her first impression, Nancy Barrand, the special advisor for program development at the Foundation, recalls him as "completely unconventional" in appearance and manner, but a riveting speaker.

The purpose of this 2001 visit was to present Foundation staff members with the results of Thomas's Eden Alternative, a precursor to Green Houses that also intended to overcome what Thomas calls the three "plagues" of nursing home life: loneliness, helplessness, and boredom.[9]

Launched in 1991, the Eden Alternative aimed at leavening the institutional feel of nursing homes by adding homelike touches such as indoor plants, pets, gardens for cultivation, and attractive and easily accessible outdoor spaces. Some nursing homes embracing Eden principles also experimented with day care centers so elderly residents could have contact with children. These tangible changes to the look and feel of nursing homes were accompanied by staff education and operational changes to encourage residents' participation in decisions about their daily routine.

A study published in 1999 by the Texas Long Term Care Institute found nursing homes that adopted Eden principles (Thomas's Eden Alternative Web site states that more than three hundred homes in the United States, Canada, Europe, and Australia participate[10]) saw decreases in the use of restraints and mood-altering drugs, improved mobility and fewer pressure sores among residents, and reduced staff absenteeism and injuries.[11] But Thomas believed the approach could be taken further, and toward the end of his presentation at the Foundation he offered up the Green House alternative: wholesale replacement of large institutional facilities with small community-based group homes.

Jane Lowe and David Colby, both Foundation senior program officers at the time, and Barrand were interested. The Foundation had considerable experience with efforts to make life easier so elderly people could remain in their homes and communities. These efforts included new ways to integrate coverage and reduce paperwork for low-income seniors who were eligible for both Medicare and Medicaid, to provide affordable housing for elderly people, and to develop home care alternatives for those who otherwise would be forced to live in a nursing home.

Colby, who now is vice president for research and evaluation, and Lowe, who currently heads the Foundation's Vulnerable Populations team, decided to do some field research to investigate Thomas's Eden accomplishments and his assertions about the state of traditional nursing homes. Accompanied by a Foundation financial officer, Colby traveled to upstate New York to see the nursing home where Thomas first tested Eden principles and to evaluate Eden principles' impact on the cost of operations. Then he and Lowe visited a traditional nursing home in Boston that was nationally renowned for its quality.

"We came out of there and both of us thought, 'Shoot me if I ever have to go into a place like that,'" Colby recalls. They returned to Princeton determined to give Thomas seed money. Barrand also was on board. "I said, 'Give him a grant,' and we ended up giving him three," she recalls.

The Foundation's first investment in Green House was a relatively modest one-year grant of $305,000 in 2002 to Thomas's Center for Growing and Becoming, in Sherburne, New York, to develop a business and development plan for Green House. Among specific tasks, Thomas was asked to create educational materials to advance the Green House organizational culture, train workers, identify technology necessary to operate a house-sized skilled nursing facility, and build a prototype for the program.

Architecturally, Green Houses mirror the overarching vision of Thomas and many others in the Pioneer Network—that people unable to live independently should still be able to reside in a place that accords dignity and respect for their abilities, interests, and life styles while also providing essential medical care and support. The dwellings are truly homelike in appearance, with private bedrooms and bathrooms, a central family room and hearth, and an adjacent open kitchen and dining area, just as one might find in a family home. At the same time, the dwellings reflect the prevailing architecture of the community, and new versions of Green Houses are in development, including a high-rise model suitable for urban areas. The first high-rise model opened in Chelsea, Massachusetts, in 2010, and another is in development in Baltimore. After all, if you've lived in an apartment all your life, a facility that looks like a suburban ranch house isn't the best substitute for home.

The food is cooked on the premises, making mealtimes not just an event on a rigid, institutional schedule marked by delivery of trays, but rather a congregating time of day signaled by bustle, kitchen clatter, and inviting aromas. Medical equipment typical of skilled nursing facilities, such as mechanized beds, medication and crash carts, and feeding tubes and oxygen jets, is deliberately tucked away in wall closets or, in the case of the beds, made up with residents' own familiar quilts, pillows, and linens. A hoist to help staff move physically disabled residents from bed to wheelchair or bathroom is hidden in bedroom ceilings and doorway arches.

Many long-term care facilities have adopted homelike touches, but Thomas and other Green House advocates assert that the scale and the organizational structure of traditional nursing homes create substantial barriers to culture change. Private rooms are rare, and staff duties are so task-oriented (for example, food service, laundry, housekeeping, transport, clinical care, therapy, social service) that it's hard for residents to form relationships. This is not the case in Green Houses, which is perhaps the model's most significant contribution to culture change.

Green Houses reverse the traditional hierarchy of staffing in nursing homes, in which those who spend the most time with residents—certified nursing assistants (CNAs)—have the least say and the least pay. This isn't a great formula for job satisfaction, as evidenced by annual industry-wide turnover rates for CNAs of 71 percent.[12] In Green Houses, the CNAs are charged with running the house in consultation with residents, nurses, other medical specialists, and a house manager, but minus the extra supervisory and administrative layers of a traditional long-term care facility. This frees up money to pay the certified nursing assistants more.

To emphasize the CNAs' enhanced hierarchical status, Thomas came up with new professional titles, semantically underscoring the break from the old ways. A CNA, who, in the Green House system receives an additional 120 hours of training, earns the title of *shahbaz,* the name of a compassionate falcon in a mythical kingdom invented by Thomas (the plural is *shahbazim*).[13] The administrator or manager of the Green House was now a "guide." And residents became "elders," echoing folkloric connotations of wisdom. These titles were of a piece with the Green House mission to support the dignity and the capabilities of residents.

"The Green House rests on a foundation of human growth and development," Thomas says. "And if that is appropriate for the elders, it is appropriate for the staff. When it works optimally, it becomes a reciprocal relationship between the staff and the elders that produces vastly more psychic income than a CNA gets operating in a traditional nursing home, and frees the creativity that's tapped from having a decision-making role in the house. Also, by eliminating the middle management structure, you free up dollars to pay [staff] better for work that goes beyond simply following orders."

—⁓— Implementing the Vision

The Robert Wood Johnson Foundation embraced Thomas's vision wholeheartedly. As presented in the Foundation's grant documents, Green Houses were an alternative to traditional nursing homes—described in these documents as "cold, sterile organizations" where seniors are "isolated from the community, lack dignity, and lose self-worth and independence." The original idea was to test the Green House concept in New York State, but the Foundation's authorization of the first grant to Thomas's Center for Growing and Becoming came on the heels of the 9/11 terrorist attacks. More than 2,700 people perished in New York City alone; in the tumultuous aftermath, obtaining the necessary approvals from health officials in New York to develop a Green House prototype proved more difficult than anticipated.

An alternate site was established in Tupelo, Mississippi, where Stephen L. McAlilly, president and CEO of Mississippi Methodist Senior Services, which owns and operates a faith-based nonprofit retirement complex, embraced the concept and made a commitment to replace its traditional nursing home with a cluster of Green Houses. In February 2003 and February 2005 the Foundation authorized two more grants to Thomas's Center for Growing and Becoming, partially to support the work in Tupelo.

Even as the Tupelo Green House was progressing, Foundation staff members say they became convinced that the Center for Growing and Becoming did not have the organizational capacity to manage national replication of the concept. Accordingly, when in November 2005 the Foundation authorized $9.5 million to expand the Green House approach nationwide, it named NCB Capital Impact as the national program office. NCB Capital, a Washington, D.C.-based organization specializing in providing financial services and technical assistance to organizations seeking to create quality housing, education, and health care services for low-income people, had gained the Foundation's trust by effectively managing an earlier Foundation-funded housing program called Coming Home. The Foundation found a willing, albeit business-minded champion for Green Houses in NCB Capital's Robert Jenkens, now the Green House national program director, whose career has focused on creating an array of alternatives to institutional nursing home care for people with low incomes. NCB Capital engaged Thomas's expertise through a contract as well as through a license agreement for use of the trademarked name Green House.

The Foundation has authorized a total of more than $12 million (including the $9.5 million in November 2005) to NCB Capital to develop a business plan, recruit and provide technical assistance to long-term care organizations around the country, and build fifty Green Houses. The program has surpassed this goal, with eighty-nine Green Houses now operating in sixteen states (see Exhibit 2.1).

Beyond supporting NCB Capital in getting the houses built and occupied, the Foundation invested an additional $500,000 in research studies. The studies, many of them still ongoing, include inquiries into psychosocial aspects of Green Houses, such as: Are residents and their families happier? Are workers? Do the small size, amenities, and staff reorientation result in improved health status among residents? And—of critical importance as the nation grapples with excessive costs and service gaps in the larger health care system—are Green Houses affordable?

"This is not just a concept for touchy-feely types," says David Morse, the Foundation's vice president for communications. "You actually have to be pretty hard-nosed about what you can do practically and what is affordable." Morse notes that views of Green House have evolved at the Foundation over nearly a decade of discussion and experimentation and that not everyone agrees. "There are still a lot of questions," he says, noting that the Foundation wants Green Houses to be an option for all elderly people, not just the well off. This means factoring in the relatively low reimbursement rates of state Medicaid programs—a challenge to Green House administrators no less than to their colleagues in traditional nursing homes.

There are also quality benchmarks for medical and supportive care that must be reached. As more Green Houses come online, providing a larger pool of residents from which to capture data, they will be put to this test. Early studies of the first Green House complex in Tupelo identified positive trends. A study published in 2006 found generally positive self-reports from residents, staff, and families, but some administrative difficulties in flattening hierarchical relationships between CNAs, registered nurses, and other clinical professionals.[14] The study concluded, "early experience suggests that Green Houses are feasible and that outcomes are likely to be positive." An evaluation published in 2007 found that Green House residents rated their overall quality of life higher than that of traditional nursing home residents, had a lower prevalence of depression, were more likely to participate in activities, and had longer retention of independent living skills such as bathing, dressing, and using the toilet. On the negative side, they had a higher prevalence of incontinence.[15] A 2009 study also found greater satisfaction among residents' families, especially with the physical environment of Green Houses and with residents' privacy and autonomy.[16]

These studies offer a generally positive initial assessment of the Green House Program, albeit one that is based on the experience of a single site in Tupelo, Mississippi. The studies identify issues that need to be explored in greater depth as more old people, families, and long-term care professionals make use of and test the Green House model. In the meantime, early adopters of the model press on. Following are two snapshots from the field.

—∿— Martin House Tabitha Health Care Services, Lincoln, Nebraska

Keith Fickenscher, the former president and chief executive officer of Tabitha Health Care Services (he left Tabitha for another position at the end of 2009), vividly remembers the initial response of his directors to the idea of building a Green House. The nonprofit health care company, which operates skilled nursing homes and provides home care, hospice services, respite care, and adult day care services, had just sunk $3.5 million into adding a rehabilitation center to its main nursing home in Lincoln—an investment that was starting to pay off, but not so heartily that Fickenscher's board was keen on more spending.

"They just kind of smiled and said, 'Well, you know it sounds nice, but it's just not practical,'" Fickenscher recalls. "It took a long time to persuade them, and there was skepticism even after they voted yes."

The result of this debate is Martin House, a graceful, red-brick one-story house on a residential street half a block from Tabitha's traditional nursing home. Built and furnished for nine residents at a cost of $1.4 million, the facility opened in May 2006, and in 2007 and 2008 generated surplus revenue over costs with six out of nine residents covered by Medicaid, according to Joyce Ebmeier, Tabitha's Green House champion and vice president of strategic planning. The company is planning construction of three more Green Houses even as it continues to work out the bugs in Thomas's theoretical model.

Most of the problems are on the operational side. The Tabitha system was already well grounded in nursing home culture change from having implemented Eden Alternative principles in 2002. But transferring these principles from an institutional setting to a small, homelike facility proved more complicated than expected, leaving staff at Martin House and management at Tabitha to fill in the gaps through trial and error.

Notably, the original model placed so much emphasis on improving certified nursing aides' status and autonomy that it gave short shrift to important operational questions such as how to integrate nurses and other specialized staff into the care team for Green House residents, most of whom were very sick. The new titles for workers—*shahbaz* and *guide*—that Thomas created to underscore the philosophical underpinnings of culture change further obscured day-to-day roles and duties, as did the emphasis on nurturing residents' autonomy, staff members say.

"The model said elders had to have a choice every morning of when they wanted to get up," says Angie Peterson, a shahbaz at Martin House and former certified nursing aide at Tabitha's traditional nursing home. "But that didn't exactly work, because we have some elders who if you gave them a choice, they'd never get out of bed, and others who'd never take a shower. We realized we had to have some structure."

Nurses say they also had to adjust the model to insure timely and appropriate clinical care of residents because it wasn't clear to shahbazim when they had to call for nursing support. The issue of nursing supervision and quality of care has come up in many Green Houses and was the focus of a Foundation-funded study by Barbara Bowers and Kim Nolet at the University of

Wisconsin-Madison School of Nursing. In a survey of eleven Green House sites, researchers found that clinical quality was not compromised by vesting greater authority in the shahbazim except in houses where nurses were seen as outsiders. In the latter case, researchers found lapses in communication of important clinical information. But in houses where the duties of shahbazim and nurses were well integrated, Bowers and Nolet concluded that clinical quality potentially was better than in traditional nursing homes. Interestingly, the study found significant differences in the shahbazim-nurse relationship from site to site and even from shift to shift.[17]

Michelle Hunter, Tabitha's director of nursing for long-term care, said she was able to compensate for deficits in the training model by handpicking nurses from the "mother ship"—a term widely used by Green House staff members to refer to the traditional nursing homes with which they're affiliated. "The staff nurses that went over to Martin House were the cream of the crop, so I knew they'd figure out how to work out the new relationships with the CNAs," Hunter says, noting that her twenty-five-year tenure at Tabitha was a great asset in selecting seasoned nurses who could adapt to the flattened hierarchy without budging on patients' clinical needs. "But as this gets bigger and we have to hire into this model, we're going to have to develop more processes for communication and divisions of responsibility."

Martin House nurses and shahbazim say they have managed to craft relationships under the Green House collaborative model to make sure no one feels either over her head or underutilized. This teamwork has led to innovations that many acknowledge would not have been possible in the rigid staff structure of a traditional nursing home. One of these innovations is an enhanced electronic medical record for each resident that shahbazim, nurses, physicians, and other specialists contribute to.

This, Hunter and others say, leads to more comprehensive and potentially better quality of care than is possible in most medical facilities where access to patient records is restricted to clinical professionals. The shahbazim's close relationships with elders enables them to contribute "rich psychosocial content" that helps an episodic worker, such as a physical therapist, understand the patient's specific needs in a broader and more humanistic context. These daily caregiver notes, particularly on patients who can't talk or who have dementia or are otherwise cognitively impaired, can also alert clinical staff to behavior changes (such as unusual fatigue, irritability, or disorientation) that can signal infection or other medical trouble in frail old people. Thomas's theory of "psychic income" plays out as well in the satisfaction shahbazim say they experience knowing they've contributed not only to elders' comfort but also to early detection of illness or injury.

Shahbazim say the Green House setting makes it easier for them to get to know residents and share their insights with fellow staffers than was possible in Tabitha's traditional nursing home, where the job emphasis was on accomplishing specific tasks—turning a bedridden patient to avoid bedsores, changing linens, assisting with personal care, and so on. These tasks are still part of the job at Green House, but the charge to shahbazim is to figure out how to work together to complete tasks efficiently so time is freed up to socialize with residents.

"I really think it helps that the elders don't have to put their trust in a hundred different employees rotating through on three shifts," says James Williams, a shahbaz who previously worked as a CNA in Tabitha's rehabilitation unit. "There are only twelve of us here at Martin House, and because the elders see us regularly, it helps them open up and feel more like a person, not just a room number."

Green Houses also smell great. No off-putting antiseptic, medicinal, or body odors here. At Martin House, visitors step into the aroma of fresh-baked chocolate chip cookies, cinnamon buns, or tangy spaghetti sauce. Recipes are often chosen for their pungency. The idea is to stimulate residents' appetites (weight loss is a significant problem in the very old) and create anticipation of a convivial gathering around the dining room table.

Videos and marketing brochures about Green House key in on these mealtime gatherings as a way to illustrate the homelike ambiance of these small-scale facilities. But staff and residents say the promotional materials tend to exaggerate the degree of interaction at meals or any other time. After all, Green Houses are licensed and reimbursed as skilled nursing facilities. Their residents suffer from the same serious physical and cognitive problems as residents of traditional nursing homes, which include stroke, dementia, swallowing, digestive and motor disorders, cancers and other acute illnesses, and chronic afflictions of the heart, lungs, liver, kidneys, and metabolism. A significant number of Green House residents cannot feed themselves or communicate well and require assistance from shahbazim or family members.

They're also, by virtue of age and infirmity, short-timers in the Green House family, which can be very hard on staff. The death of a beloved resident—one of the first to die at Martin House—revealed significant deficits in the preparation of shahbazim for losing people they'd been trained to bond with so personally. Reacting protectively, as is their duty under the Green House model, shahbazim closed the house to new admissions for an indefinite period of mourning, recalls Fickenscher, Tabitha's former president and CEO.

"I'm hearing this as an administrator who knows the finances don't allow for unfilled beds," Fickenscher says. "It really surprised a lot of us, and it took a lot of explaining to persuade them that to stay viable we have to do some things that may not seem too sensitive but they're necessary. It was a very tough situation."

The experience illuminated the need for hospice-type training as part of the orientation for new shahbazim, according to Jeremy Hohlen, Martin House's guide. There's now also a "celebration of life" ceremony with refreshments, spontaneous storytelling, and even PowerPoint slide shows to mark an elder's passing—and clear the way for a new resident. Harsh as that may sound, Green Houses are businesses no less than nursing homes. This aspect of long-term care facility management is harder to disguise in a small, homelike setting than in a large institution.

On an evening last fall, Martin House residents and shahbazim gathered for dinner and welcomed some visitors to their table, among them Gregg Wright, a physician and former director of the Nebraska Department of Health, who had stopped by after work to visit his ninety-seven-year-old mother, Marian, one of Martin House's first residents when it opened in 2006. Marian Wright initially was in the middle of the group in terms of independence, according to her son, but now she's one of the most disabled. As his mother slumps in her wheelchair, eyes half-closed, Wright gently strokes her hand and tries to coax her into swallowing a spoonful of pudding.

Across the table is Margaret Hall, wheelchair-bound but fully able to handle her own knife and fork and converse amiably with residents and visitors alike. For most of her adult life, Hall worked as a librarian in Chicago, serving on the prestigious Newbery Medal committee of the American Library Association. She was a committee member when the novel *Charlotte's Web*, by E.B. White—destined to become a classic of children's literature—was nominated for the prize. "I voted for it—I didn't think any other nominee even came close," Hall recounts. "But I was in the minority and the medal went to another book."

Hall continues to be an avid reader and participates in the house book group, which sounds like just the sort of resident-sponsored activity Green Houses were conceived to nurture. But the book group's organizer, former schoolteacher Helen "Mike" Holmes, eighty-three, says her experience has been disappointing, illuminating a downside of small group living; it is difficult to find companions with similar interests and abilities.

"We haven't been able to get very far with everyone reading the same book," says Holmes, who'd just finished a biography of Eleanor Roosevelt and wished she had someone to discuss it with.

"People forget to show up or when they do they haven't read the book or didn't like it so just quit reading. So now we just read our own book and share the stories if enough people show up for a meeting."

Holmes, though, is quick to put these observations in context, namely her decided preference for Martin House in favor of the life she had at Tabitha. She cites amenities like private rooms and bathrooms as well as greater personal freedom.

"I was on the second floor over there in the nursing home and my care plan said I couldn't go outside without an attendant," she says. "But now when the weather's good, I just wheel myself outside anytime I want. I can read on the patio or on the front porch all day long."

Family members like Greg Wright significantly extend the appreciative constituency of Green Houses. Indeed, they may be the model's strongest proponents—even after their loved ones have passed on. Zoe Holland still visits Martin House from time to time in gratitude for her late mother's experience there.

Holland has testified on behalf of the Green House model before the Senate's Special Committee on Aging,[18] eloquently describing the contrast between the four years her mother Mary Valentine spent in a traditional nursing home and her final year in Martin House. Valentine died three weeks after a grand 101st birthday party at the house, but during the year she spent there, recovered the spirit she'd lost sharing a cramped nursing home room with only a curtain for privacy and no place for personal mementos. And Holland says her own spirits rebounded with her mother's.

"We dreaded going to the nursing home to visit; the environment was just so depressing," Holland recalls. "But at Martin House, we could visit my mother in her room or on the porch or in the living room. Granddaughter Liz could play the violin for the whole house where before, at the nursing home, she had to play standing in the hall—the room was that small!

"Once I could see that my mother was happy and secure in the Green House, it was easier for my husband and me to travel, knowing we could call anytime and talk to caregivers who really knew her. The value of that peace of mind is hard to overstate."

—⁓— Eddy Village Green Northeast Health, Cohoes, New York

Like her administrative counterparts at Tabitha, Jo-Ann Costantino, executive vice president of Northeast Health in upstate New York, had a bushel of logistical and financial variables to sort through before she could commit to constructing Green Houses. Scale was the overriding variable.

Northeast Health is like Tabitha in that it operates many health care businesses besides long-term care facilities. Northeast Health also ranges more widely than Tabitha, running hospitals, rehabilitation services, and primary care facilities, in addition to nursing homes and other services for the elderly. Its territory covers twenty-two counties surrounding the state capital of Albany. Its long-term care network is known as "The Eddy" after the founder of its first nursing home, Elizabeth Hart Shields Eddy.

The Green House proposal dovetailed with an urgent need for renovation of two traditional nursing homes located at The Eddy's complex in Cohoes, New York. "Basically we had twenty-five- to thirty-year-old buildings that needed $25 million in repairs—plumbing, electric, everything," says Costantino, who is also chief executive officer of the Eddy. For an estimated $40 million, The Eddy could construct a village of Green Houses, move in the nursing home residents, and tear down the old buildings. This is the route The Eddy eventually chose, albeit with significant modifications to the Green House model. When completed, Eddy Village Green will feature sixteen ranch houses for twelve residents each, for a total of 192 skilled nursing beds. Laurie Mante, The Eddy's project manager, says the facilities' small size makes them easy to adapt to the clinical needs of a wide range of people—a flexibility that's important in the ever-shifting health care market and that helps justify The Eddy's construction investment.

"We're a nonprofit organization, but we have an obligation to operate in a fiscally sound manner," Costantino says. "What I'm saying is I'm not taking a bath on an idea, however appealing, that can't be justified by the numbers."

Bumping up the number of residents from ten (the optimal number for Green Houses, according to Thomas) to twelve was the first change to the model. "We simply couldn't make ten work financially," Costantino says. (Ten residents is the maximum for use of the trademarked Green House name, except in cases of demonstrated hardship, according to Jenkens, the national program director.) Staff training also differs from the original model, thanks in part to test runs by early adopters like Tabitha. The first houses at Eddy Village Green opened in December 2008, more than two years after Tabitha's Martin House. Administrators attended educational sessions offered by the Green House national program office, but also visited the Tupelo project and consulted with frontline workers and managers elsewhere.

As a result, shahbazim and nurses at Eddy Village have been trained together from day one—and there's no fuzziness about their mutual and separate responsibilities. "We saw a concept that went so far out of its way to elevate the shahbazim that it made the nurses outsiders," says Diana Lloyd, director of nursing. "What we basically said about the model on this point is, 'You blew it.' Shahbazim have twelve extra days of training over traditional certified nursing assistants, which is very laudable, but it does not qualify them to do nursing work or make licensed practical nurse- or registered nurse-level clinical judgments."

To delineate when shahbazim must hand off responsibility to nurses, Lloyd devised a two-hour course to help shahbazim recognize so-called emergent clinical situations requiring immediate medical response. The shahbazim are also equipped with call pendants; if one of them pushes the button, the nearest nurse must drop everything and rush to her aid.

Another departure from the model is the higher nurse–resident ratio at Eddy Village—an adaptation to what administrators believe are sicker residents than at other sites experimenting with Green Houses. Most of the experimental sites function as satellites of traditional nursing homes and share the same campus. This enables them to be selective in who qualifies for the Green House. Eddy Village, in contrast, is designed to be freestanding with no institutional backup. Already, 85 percent of the elders in the sixteen completed houses have dementia, and some houses have no patients who are able to walk on their own or feed themselves or talk, according to Cheryll Schampier, guide (manager) of three of the houses. This contrast between the promotional image of Green Houses as convivial, interactive communities and the manifest acuity of illness and disability at Eddy Village fired up debate when a production company sought permission to film at Eddy Village for a video about Green Houses. "Across the board, the feedback from staff was, 'OK, but not if they're just going to focus on residents who can talk and smile for the camera," said Lloyd.

Shahbaz Tracy Price agrees the inspirational Green House message can obscure the reality of this final stage of life. The first resident under her care died three days after arriving in the house. "It is not the utopia that they try to sell it as," Price says. "We have elders with all kinds of personalities, attitudes, problems, and psychological states. It's hard some days, and not everyone can be happy."

But Price, a one-time nursing student who shifted to shahbaz training because of its emphasis on "hands-on personal caring," also sees many pluses in the small-scale environment and many opportunities to be creative. "We have found that intergenerational mixing delights the elders," she says. "My kids sometimes stop by to visit me here after school and the elders all know them. Pets are also very big. And we also see progress, which is very rewarding. A new resident came in with late-stage Alzheimer's who we were told didn't talk. Well, after a month here, she was talking."

—∿— **Conclusion**

Stanley Radzyminski is matter-of-fact about the circumstances that made it impossible for him and his late wife Edna to continue to live independently in their home. He accepts this stoically, with the understanding of every Green House resident interviewed for this chapter that their best years are most definitely behind them. There's not a lot of talk about happiness or personal growth and development. Residents' conversations tend to be about practical concerns and tangible, even if small, successes.

For Radzyminski, a success was getting the Green House staff to rearrange the furniture in his and Edna's assigned rooms so they could continue to share a bedroom and convert the other bedroom to a parlor. For Holmes, a success was being able to roll her wheelchair out onto the patio without needing permission or an attendant. For Eddy Village resident Frederick Britting, ninety-six, it's the relief of having a private room after sharing one "at the big house" with a man whose wife hollered and threatened divorce every time she came to visit.

Because Green Houses are still relatively new, most of their current residents previously lived in traditional nursing homes. The elders' comparisons are strikingly judicious in contrast to the rhetoric of nursing home reformers like Thomas. Green House residents go out of their way to point out that their nursing home caregivers were good people, too, and some mention advantages of the large facilities such as more activities and a greater variety of people.

To position Green Houses as radically different from nursing homes, Thomas invented new language and a mythological story line to inspire nursing home workers to think differently about their jobs. He gave new titles and authority to frontline workers and special training to imbue them with a sense of mission. The idea of improving residents' lives by increasing monetary and psychic rewards for the people most involved in their care seems like Management 101, except that virtually no one did anything about the industry's shocking CNA turnover rate until Bill Thomas came along.

That said, evidence from the Green House field suggests that the long-term care reform movement would benefit from plainer speech about the realities of frail old age. Decisions at Eddy Village and Martin House to more closely integrate nurses into the care team were forced by deficiencies in a staff training model that failed to adequately account for the severity of illness and disability in people who require skilled nursing care. Additional training is now being done. "I think we underestimated how important it was to also train nurses to work in a Green House environment because we had changed so many elements of the traditional nursing home organizational model," says NCB Capital's Robert Jenkens.

Green House sites continue to work through operational issues such as these, while also keeping a close eye on costs so Green Houses can remain an option for people dependent upon Medicaid.

The Green House concept is unquestionably an attractive one, and there is sure to be push from families of the frail elderly attracted by the appeal of a homelike setting where an aged parent can receive sophisticated medical care and social support. Moreover, the long-term care industry has shown itself to be receptive to innovation, especially now as it girds itself for major investments to replace or remodel deteriorating facilities while also expanding capacity to prepare for baby boomers.

Time will tell, however, whether Green Houses and other congregate living models replace more institutional nursing homes or exist alongside them as one of many residential care options. Better knowledge about clinical, operational, and financial results from studies of Green House and other reform experiments will provide much-needed anchors for long-term care policy.

Appendix: The Green House® Project Site Map

THE GREEN HOUSE® Project is a project of NCB Capital Impact and is funded by the Robert Wood Johnson Foundation.

Notes

1. Centers for Disease Control and Prevention, National Center for Health Statistics. "Nursing Home Care." *Fastats.* http://www.cdc.gov/nchs/fastats/nursingh.htm.

2. Kaiser Family Foundation. "Update on the Public's Views of Nursing Homes and Long-Term Care Services." *Kaiser Public Opinion Spotlight.* Kaiser Family Foundation Survey, October 1–10, 2007. http://www.kff.org/spotlight/longterm/index.cfm.

3. Harrington, C., Carrillo, H., and Blank, B.W. *Nursing Facilities, Staffing, Residents and Facility Deficiencies, 2003 through 2008.* Department of Social and Behavioral Sciences, University of California, San Francisco, November 2009.

4. Institute of Medicine, Committee on Nursing Home Regulation. *Improving the Quality of Care in Nursing Homes.* Washington, D.C.: National Academies Press, 1986.

5. Jones, L. *Great Expectations: America and the Baby Boom Generation.* New York: Coward, McCann & Geoghegan, 1980.

6. U. S. Census Bureau. *Selected Characteristics of Baby Boomers 42 to 60 Years Old in 2006.* 2006. http://www.census.gov/population/www/socdemo/age/2006%20Baby%20Boomers.pdf.

7. U.S. Administration on Aging. *A Profile of Older Americans, 2009.* 2009. http://www.aoa.gov/AoARoot/Aging_Statistics/future_growth/future_growth.aspx#age.

8. Administration on Aging, Department of Health and Human Services. *Understanding Long-Term Care: Definitions and Risks.* 2008. http://www.longtermcare.gov/LTC/Main_Site/Understanding_Long_Term_Care/Basics/Basics.aspx.

9. Eden Alternative. *About the Eden Alternative.* 2009. http://www.edenalt.org/about-the-eden-alternative.

10. Ibid.

11. Eden Alternative. *1999 Statistical Report Summary of Eden Alternative Outcomes in Texas.* 2000. http://www.edenalt.org/images/stories/newsletter/research/1999_statistics_summary.pdf.

12. American Association of Homes and Services for the Aged. *Aging Services: The Facts.* http://www.aahsa.org/article.aspx?id=74.

13. Thomas, W. H. *What Are Old People For? How Elders Will Save the World.* Acton, Mass.: VanderWyk & Burnham, 2004.

14. Rabig, J., and others. "Radical Redesign of Nursing Homes: Applying the Green House Concept in Tupelo, Mississippi." *The Gerontologist,* 2006, *46*, 533–539.

15. Kane, R., and others. "Resident Outcomes in Small-House Nursing Homes: A Longitudinal Evaluation of the Initial Green House Program." *Journal of the American Geriatrics Society,* 2007, *55,* 832–839.

16. Lum, T. Y., and others. "Effects of Green House Nursing Homes on Residents' Families." *Health Care Financing Review,* 2008–2009, *30*(2), 35–51.

17. Bowers, B., and Nolet, K. *Exploring the Role of the Nurse in Implementing the Green House Model.* University of Wisconsin, unpublished research study, 2010.

18. Testimony of Zoe Valentine Holland, hearing before the Special Committee on Aging. U.S. Senate, Washington, D. C., July 23, 2008.

CHAPTER 3

Playworks/Sports4Kids

Carolyn Newbergh

Editors' Introduction

Good ideas emerge from all kinds of unexpected places. In this chapter, Carolyn Newbergh, a California-based freelance journalist who has contributed many chapters to the *Anthology* series, tells the story of a promising program that emerged from a conversation between an activist trying to raise money for a children's art museum and an Oakland elementary school principal who, concerned about making recess less unruly, asked why nobody was doing anything about bringing play back onto the playground.

Activist Jill Vialet took the question as a challenge, and from it she developed the idea of Playworks—originally called Sports4Kids. Playworks brings young adults, many of them AmeriCorps volunteers, to schools in low-income urban communities, where they organize and oversee recess periods and sometimes after-school activities. The idea behind Playworks, as Vialet expresses it, is to bring play back into the lives of America's children. With support from the Robert Wood Johnson Foundation, Sports4Kids expanded from a pilot project in a handful of San Francisco Bay Area schools to a national program, Playworks, that has received nearly universal accolades from students, teachers, parents, and the media.

There is, however, a cloud on the horizon: whether a program such as this—which benefits disadvantaged children and generates tremendous enthusiasm in most places it is tried—is affordable in hard economic times. School districts throughout the nation are being forced to make the difficult decision about whether to spend the more than $20,000 a year this program costs them. In this regard, the chapter on Playworks/Sports4Kids is more than the story of a program that provides supervised play for vulnerable school children. It is also a case study of the challenges inherent in sustaining programs, even ones acknowledged to have great promise.

Not long ago, the playground at Manzanita Community School in Oakland was emblematic of all that has gone wrong with recess in the United States, especially in low-income neighborhoods. Because of concerns about lawsuits, monkey bars and other play structures had been removed. Meanwhile, much of the play equipment, from the jump ropes to the hula hoops, had gone missing. Students faced a sea of blacktop when they headed out to recess. They knew how to do only a few things—kick a ball as far as they could and hope someone might kick it back, punch a tetherball, or pile onto the lone play structure and elbow and shove one another as they climbed or sat on it. It was aimless play, and only a fraction of the students joined in. Mostly they fought over who could use the ball, called names, bullied, gossiped, pushed, and shoved. Many of the pupils, especially the girls, clung to the sidelines, with no interest in participating in the chaotic and often intimidating scene. Injuries on the playground were common, and bad behavior led to disciplinary referrals to the principal and to suspensions.

Each day, the students at this elementary school would return to class from recess riled up, distracted, and unable to concentrate. Teachers wasted precious learning time calming the children down. The tone of the school was "like the wild West," with children willfully walking out of classrooms when they felt like it, slamming doors, and toting BB guns to school, said Eyana Spencer, the school's principal.

Beginning in the 2005–2006 school year, Manzanita introduced a new approach to managing recess, outsourcing it to Sports4Kids, a nonprofit Oakland-based program that took the name Playworks in 2009. A high-energy young coach taught the schoolchildren how to play a range of basic childhood games they either didn't know the rules for or had never learned, such as hopscotch, four square, double Dutch jump rope, kickball, switch, and much more. The emphasis was on having fun, not playing to win at all costs—and on including everyone. The coach, a young, college-educated adult brimming with enthusiasm, became the star of the playground, orchestrating activities at various stations on the blacktop during recess and lunch, teaching new games to the children in their classrooms, and overseeing after-school activities and leagues. He also gave the children a tool for resolving conflicts by themselves rather than in response to a teacher's angry commands, using the old children's hand game of rock-paper-scissors, which is also called *roshambo*. The school paid Sports4Kids $23,500 a year for the program, and Sports4Kids picked up the rest of the $55,000 to $60,000 tab.

On a recent autumn day, the students bounded onto the blacktop, running to various stations in the play yard. At the jump rope section, the rope circled round and round to the old standard jingle, "Ice cream soda, cherry on the top, who's your boyfriend? I forgot." Shrieks of laughter filled the air as others on the playground played dodgeball, basketball, and four square. Some children waited in line to check out equipment from *junior coaches*—older students the Playworks coach had chosen to be peer leaders on the playground.

Suddenly a dispute erupted. A child who was up next to turn the rope walked away, and the children angrily yelled at him, "You have to tell us you're leaving, because it was your turn." Quickly, the Sports4Kids coach, Jared Crayton-Thomas, explained that rule and reminded the children to use rock-paper-scissors to resolve the disagreement. A few moments later, the boy picked up the rope and joined in the fun. Tranquility was restored.

"It's nothing short of amazing," said Haydee Jimenez, who has had three children at the school, one of them a former junior coach. "All this order and good behavior and respect—it wasn't anything like this a couple of years ago. Oh my goodness, there used to be a lot of fights and bullies."

Manzanita, a long-troubled school that was reconstituted in 2005 to improve the learning environment, has seen remarkable results from Playworks, said principal Spencer, who handpicked its teachers and insisted that Sports4Kids be invited in. Since then, suspensions have dropped, test scores have edged up some, and teachers report that they no longer lose a major chunk of class time to the spillover of unhappiness from recess. The students treat one another and their teachers with more respect, and the tone of the campus has improved, she said.

"The climate of our school changed with Sports4Kids, because there is another caring adult on campus who can help the kids and keep the playground safe for them," Spencer says. "Jared motivates the kids, engages with them, and the kids have fun together. It helps children to have a good connection with someone they play with when they're a partner with that person later in the day in math."

—ᴡ— The Decline of Recess and Play

Sports4Kids, now Playworks, started out in 1996 as the brainchild of Jill Vialet, a woman who is often called a visionary. She took a principal's off-the-cuff cry for help with recess and has turned its solution into a national movement, with the help of a $29 million investment by the Robert Wood Johnson Foundation that has propelled the organization's expansion.

Vialet built the nonprofit program in eighty San Francisco Bay Area schools, bringing "safe and healthy" play to 32,000 children for ten years, and then, together with support from the Robert Wood Johnson Foundation, set in motion a plan to expand the program to 650 schools in twenty-seven cities—directly reaching 260,000 children and indirectly touching thousands more through its training and technical assistance. With support from the Foundation, Sports4Kids set out to lead a movement to recognize, at a time when play and recess are shortchanged in favor of efforts to improve academic performance, that play and recess have a critical role in child development and must be part of every child's school day.

"The case for creative and constructive play is a compelling one," said Risa Lavizzo-Mourey, president and chief executive officer of the Robert Wood Johnson Foundation. "It's good for kids' development of social skills and learning how to mediate differences and how to learn to make rules that they can live by and play by. It has the added benefit of being absolutely consistent with one of our key strategic objectives, to reverse childhood obesity. Over time, kids have to get more physically active, and one of the untapped times for that is recess. When you put all of those things together, it is compelling to try to fix the lack of opportunity many kids have to play."

The urgency behind the push for a movement stemmed from the downward spiral of both recess and play, especially in low-income and minority urban communities. Nationwide, recess has been getting shorter or eliminated as schools focus on bringing up math, reading, and science test scores under federal No Child Left Behind mandates and struggle with mounting financial pressures. The National Parent Teacher Association stated in 2006 that "nearly 40 percent of American elementary schools have either eliminated or are considering eliminating recess."[1] The Center for Public Education, an initiative of the National School Boards Association, found in a 2007 survey that 20 percent of school districts had reduced the time they allocated for recess in response to No Child Left Behind.[2] Meanwhile, although many states require schools to provide a minimum amount of physical activity, most do not monitor whether the stretched-thin schools comply.

Olga Jarrett, a recess advocate and researcher who is an associate professor of early childhood education at Georgia State University, found in a study on fourth graders that they were "more fidgety and less on task" on days they did not have recess.[3] "They had less focus in terms of making eye contact with a teacher, working with a classmate on a project, reading, or filling out a worksheet," said Jarrett, who is also president of the American Association for the Child's Right to Play. "They were less apt to be doing what they were supposed to be doing when they didn't have recess."

Recess would not be so critical if children were getting enough play time outside of school, but many factors have conspired to reduce the opportunities for normal childhood physical play. What kids used to pick up by apparent osmosis from older siblings or neighborhood kids is no longer so common in childhood. In the old days, children returned home after school and drew a hopscotch grid on their driveway or sidewalk or flew out of their front doors to ride bikes with friends in the neighborhood. Now busy working parents tell their kids to stay inside at home after school. There is little of the merry sound of kids bouncing balls, skipping rope, or playing four square during the afternoon in low-income urban neighborhoods. Too many children are indoors watching TV or playing video games—sedentary, individual pursuits with little social interaction or physical movement—and that feeds the childhood obesity epidemic. Children from low-income families face other barriers to leading active lifestyles. They cannot, for example, afford to join after-school sports leagues or to take ballet, martial arts, or other enriching lessons. Meanwhile, in the inner cities, they may be exposed to violence, shootings, and drug dealing while peeking out the living room curtains, afraid to go outside.

"Child's play" may sound frivolous and unimportant, but experts say it is anything but—that play matters and must be taken seriously. Without it, children don't develop important skills they will need throughout life. A 2007 American Academy of Pediatrics report described play as "essential to development because it contributes to the cognitive, physical, social, and emotional well-being of children and youth." Play is "important to healthy brain development" and should be integrated into the academic day, the report said. Play "ensures that the school setting attends to the social and emotional development of children as well as their cognitive development. It has been shown to help children adjust to the school setting, and even to enhance children's learning readiness, learning behaviors, and problem-solving skills."[4] A 2009 Yeshiva University study of 11,000 third graders concluded that giving children a recess break of at least fifteen minutes a day improved their behavior and left them more likely to learn.[5]

─᠊᠊᠊᠊ The Result of a Casual Conversation

Playworks sprang from a casual conversation in 1995. Seated on one of those short elementary school chairs, Vialet was waiting to speak to an Oakland school principal, Margaret Peyton, about a children's art museum Vialet had founded. Three fifth-grade boys who had fought during recess trudged out of Peyton's office, tails between their legs. While meeting with Vialet, the principal praised the museum but lamented that she had her hands full with kids who misbehave during recess. "She said that these were not bad kids but they're starting to believe they're bad kids," Vialet recalled. "She was so agitated and said, 'Can't you do something about *this?*'"

Peyton's distress planted a seed in Vialet, who thought back to her own childhood in Washington, D.C. A sports-loving kid, Vialet tended to be the only girl who wanted to play some games—but the boys often wouldn't let her participate. It took the intervention and advocacy of the playground coordinator from the local parks and recreation department, whom she refers to as Clarence, to break down barriers for her to play. She wondered if what was missing on school playgrounds today was a Clarence—someone to watch out for the kids, smooth out the discord, and show them how to have fun.

Vialet decided to try an experiment at Columbus [now Rosa Parks] and Cragmont elementary schools in Berkeley, hiring and training a part-time site coordinator who would act as a game supervisor and coach to teach kids the how-to's and rules of games like four square and dodgeball. The coordinator taught that the goal of play was not to vanquish your opponent but to have fun and play cooperatively. No one was to be left out of the games. "We wanted a culture in which you didn't want to crush the other side—rather, you wanted the other side to want to play with you," Vialet said. "If it's not fun for everyone, they wouldn't play." The site coordinators didn't just oversee the playground but played the games alongside the children and encouraged teachers to join in also. This way, kids could observe their teachers having fun, too, and teachers could see their pupils in a different light.

The Berkeley Public Education Foundation, a private non-profit that supported the schools, contributed $5,000 to the experiment. "The kids responded so well," said Mary Friedman, who headed the fund at the time. "Children love structure and being told what to do, particularly when it's fun and it's on the playground. It takes away that free-floating anxiety of not knowing what to do. We had lots of happy faces."

It was quickly clear that Vialet was on to something, and in the second year the program expanded to five schools in Oakland, with financial support from the private Evelyn and Walter Haas, Jr. Fund and the citizen-supported Oakland Fund for Children and Youth. It opened its offices in a converted warehouse in downtown Oakland and began employing full-time coaches and choosing junior coaches from among the older school children to pitch in as peer leaders—teaching games, resolving disputes, and checking out equipment. The junior coaches were either some of the more responsible, high-achieving students or some of those who were struggling but might benefit from being given responsibility and higher expectations. Rock-paper-scissors would be key to resolving conflicts, giving children a tool that allowed them to move on from disagreement. "Rock-paper-scissors is a strategy to solve any conflict, every time," said Vialet, a Harvard graduate who played rugby while in college. "Kids are able to move on. They want to keep playing, and this gives them a strategy to keep playing."

In its third year, the organization continued to expand, and it also gave the site coordinators the task of leading an after-school program. By increasing the responsibilities of the coach position, the program was able to offer coaches full-time jobs with health insurance. After school, coaches oversaw homework help, a healthy snack, and sports and games until 5:00 P.M. In an effort to encourage girls to participate in sports, Sports4Kids started an interscholastic athletic league for girls in fourth and fifth grades.

In 2002, Sports4Kids began a partnership with the California branch of AmeriCorps, the national youth service program, which provided a pipeline of idealistic, energetic young volunteers fresh out of college, along with substantial financial assistance and stability.

As it expanded to eighty schools in the San Francisco Bay Area during its first ten years, much about this program was fine-tuned. Sports4Kids tried different approaches to calculating a fee, arriving at $23,500 per school annually—about half the cost of a first-year teacher's salary. This covered 40 percent of the program's cost, and Sports4Kids picked up the remaining 60 percent in each city through grants from foundations, government support, and contributions from private donors. Each school had its own coach, who was on-site all day to run recess, meet with each classroom teacher, and oversee junior coaches and the after-school program. The organization developed a rigorous training program on games and managing conflict and developed extensive curriculum materials so that coaches were well prepared when they hit the blacktop. The program documented its approaches to assure consistency and see that new staff members wouldn't have to reinvent the wheel.

By 2005, this feisty organization (many in the Oakland office wore shorts to work) with a $2.94 million annual budget was ready to move beyond the San Francisco Bay Area. In the spring of that year, the Robert Wood Johnson Foundation approached Vialet with the idea of expanding Sports4Kids to schools in low-income communities throughout the country. While negotiations were proceeding, Sports4Kids ventured into Baltimore, where some school principals had been clamoring for the program. "What we were doing locally was resonating nationally, we discovered," Vialet said. "When Baltimore took off, we thought that there was clearly demand everywhere."

—∿— The Robert Wood Johnson Foundation Gets Involved

Vialet and Sports4Kids had come to the Foundation's attention through Bill Drayton, a man who pioneered the concept of *social entrepreneurs*—innovators who bring solutions to pressing social problems through transformative change. Drayton founded Ashoka, an international organization that supports social entrepreneurs; Vialet was an Ashoka Fellow in 2004. Invited to speak at the Robert Wood Johnson Foundation, Drayton suggested Vialet's Sports4Kids as a good fit for the Foundation because of its commitment to eliminating childhood obesity. "We predicted she would change the pattern [of physical activity at schools] across the country at least," Drayton said in an interview. "Now it's five years later and I think it's pretty clear that she is going to do that."

As part of its Vulnerable Populations portfolio of grants, the Foundation approached Sports4Kids about expanding. "We were looking at the time for innovative community-based models that could be scaled up and replicated," said Nancy Barrand, the Foundation's special adviser for program development. The idea was to bring to more children a program that would improve their well-being, promote their physical activity, and enhance their learning environment. It was not envisioned as an obesity-prevention program per se, although any venture that increased exercise among children would certainly help reduce obesity.

The Foundation asked Vialet to think about what it would take to expand the program across the country. She and the

Foundation arrived at a plan to continue the program's expansion in Baltimore and replicate it in Boston and Washington, D.C., under a three-year $4.4 million grant that would run through June 2008. The grant would help cover Sports4Kids' share of expenses for expanding to about sixty new schools and the costs of building a national office staff in Oakland to support the larger operation. As a result, $400,000 was earmarked for communications.

Barrand recalls the program as a fairly easy sell at the Foundation. "This is all about how to use the power of play, the leverage of play, the momentum behind the fact that children like to play to accomplish certain goals—to increase physical activity, learn rules, learn conflict resolution, be better able to sit in class and focus more," she said. "It was a very different approach, perhaps accomplishing things more directly than other programs of ours."

The partnership with the Robert Wood Johnson Foundation started in 2005. In community organizer mode, Vialet set out, armed with research on who the star local principals were, the ones interested in trying innovative programs and taking risks. She would drop in on them unannounced, talk up the program, and explore their ability to use federal Title I funds to cover the school's portion of the cost, which most were able to do. (Funding from Title I of the Elementary and Secondary Education Act is available to schools with low-achieving students living in high-poverty areas.) Sports4Kids would perform a one-week demonstration for the schools on how the program worked and on what it could do for them. Nearly always, the principals, teachers, and kids were dazzled by the infusion of energy, discipline, and fun.

The Robert Wood Johnson funding not only covered much of the cost of expanding but also acted as a stamp of legitimacy that attracted potential donors in the three cities, opening doors to establish relationships critical to raising the additional money the program needed. It helped Sports4Kids attain important support from the national AmeriCorps and from local AmeriCorps organizations in the states beginning in 2007. By 2009, AmeriCorps accounted for 10 percent of the Sports4Kids annual budget.

Sports4Kids played out in the three new cities as it had in Northern California. Teachers, principals, and parents were thrilled that the horror time of recess was now transformed to a period that was orderly and fun, and the school's learning atmosphere improved. "There was a lot of word of mouth, people talking about schools that had it, and I wanted in," said Mary Donnelly, principal of John Ruhrah Elementary in Baltimore. "It was a really nice program—the kids and the principals loved it. I loved seeing everyone engaged."

Eileen Nash, a principal for two Boston schools, observed remarkable changes on the campuses, noting that the junior coach piece of the program encouraged some troublemaking kids to straighten out. "A couple of tough kids became junior coaches," she said. "The kids live and die to wear the purple T-shirts of the junior coach. They got to succeed and feel really good about helping the younger kids with four square. It is amazing to see what it does for these kids' self esteem."

And at Washington, D.C.'s Brookland Education Campus @ Bunker Hill, principal Donna Pressley watched in wonder as the play yard that had seemed impossible to organize became orderly. "Recess has become popular again," Pressley said. "It translates wonderfully in the classroom, and has helped our overall school climate. Now nobody wants to lose time playing, so they make sure to cooperate and work hard."

—∞— Assessing the Program

The expansion into Boston brought with it an unanticipated benefit—a Harvard Graduate School of Education program studied the impact that Sports4Kids had on one of the local schools, William H. Ohrenberger Elementary in West Roxbury, during the 2006–2007 school year. The report, titled *Evaluation Report: Case Study of the First Year of Sports4Kids at the Ohrenberger Elementary School,* confirmed what principals, teachers, and parents had been saying for years. The report concluded, "Sports4Kids helped youth to feel safe on the playground and in the classroom. In addition, we saw some evidence that Sports4Kids contributed to a more positive academic environment for youth. Specifically, when youth have a productive outlet for their physical energy, they are better able to focus in the classroom, which in turn promotes better academic performance. While this alone is unlikely to translate into higher test scores or better grades, Sports4Kids may be one factor that contributes to improved academic performance."[6]

A report by the University of California, Berkeley, *Sports4Kids Cumulative Report,* on the program in ten Bay Area schools during the 2007–2008 school year reached similar positive conclusions. The number of children who were overweight declined 1 percent, and there was a 13 percent improvement in aerobic capacity among fifth graders. Both changes were statistically significant.[7] The students largely enjoyed the program. In the one-third of schools in which students were less engaged in the program, the study's authors suggested this may be explained by how Sports4Kids was implemented in those schools, by particular "student characteristics" in the schools, or by other variables. "The improvements seen in students' weight status and fitness suggest that Sports4Kids has a positive impact on student health outcomes through increased opportunities for meaningful play," wrote the authors.

At the same time, individual schools reported that Sports4Kids was indeed improving student behavior. For example, a San Jose principal noted that suspensions had declined from forty-one to fourteen in the year since the program began. "While I can't say that adding Sports4Kids is the sole reason, the impact that organized games and responsible behavior toward one another has on our students is evident," wrote Lisa Marie Gonzalez, principal of the Bachrodt Academy.

Meanwhile, Sports4Kids received generally glowing news coverage. For example, in a story headlined "Program Helps City Kids Learn to be Good Sports: Conflict Resolution Plan Seen as Factor in Lowering Suspensions," Debbie D. Thomas, principal of Medfield Heights Elementary in Baltimore, told *The Baltimore Sun,* "We had some students who were very explosive. But they have calmed down. I've seen the difference." And a *Sun* editorial praised Sports4Kids: "One model program, in use at 11 Baltimore schools, has shown that fitness and play can be provided at a reasonable cost, with minimum equipment.... It's a good way to allow kids to let off steam, have some fun and get some exercise—all at the same time."

—⌇— Growing Pains

But Sports4Kids also found that expansion came with growing pains, that there were challenges both expected and unexpected, and that adjustments would need to be made as lessons were learned. The program ran into serious cash flow problems, because the $1.5 million line of credit that had been adequate for covering expenses while Sports4Kids waited for schools to make their fee payments was insufficient once the number of schools served grew. (Schools typically pay fees monthly, and when schools were in arrears, Sports4Kids had to carry the costs until they paid.) In 2007, cash flow reached a crisis point, sending the program scrambling until it found a savior, a Texas donor who provided an additional line of credit. Even so, it was a time of high anxiety.

The expansion created turmoil and rebellion within the informal and committed Sports4Kids culture, with many staff and board members concerned the organization was losing its soul and distrustful of Vialet and the Robert Wood Johnson Foundation. These dissenters felt the expansion was being driven by the Foundation and questioned whether the program should be growing beyond its original scope at all. The upshot was that many of those who disagreed with the new direction left.

The move beyond the Bay Area, with all of its needs for increased staffing and support, also revealed that this scrappy organization—which had tended to promote from within—lacked some of the expertise needed to handle the complexity of running a large organization. Many longtime employees were wearing multiple hats and some of them did not have the skills needed for their new roles. As a result, Sports4Kids created new positions and recruited people to handle human resources, information technology, quality, and finances.

The program also found that its directors in the three East Coast cities needed more support, and area director and officer manager positions were added. It was no longer enough for one person to function alone in each city as Vialet had done in the beginning in Oakland. What's more, the role of Vialet herself, who was overextended, was narrowed, and in 2008, Sports4Kids hired an executive director, David Rothenberg, to manage the organization's daily operations. Vialet remained as president, acting as the strategic leader, national spokesperson, and leading national fundraiser.

—ᴧᴧ— Expanding Nationwide

In 2008, with the program in place at 131 schools, Sports4Kids, with Robert Wood Johnson Foundation support, took the program to scale. A four-year $17 million grant enabled Sports4Kids to serve 260,000 children at 650 schools in twenty-seven cities and to serve thousands more schools through a fee-charging technical assistance and training program for parents, teachers, and others interested in incorporating the Sports4Kids approach. Sports4Kids envisioned leading a movement for play in schools. "We are working to get enough geographic presence that we become the gold standard and to some extent a household word," Vialet said. "So when people hear 'Playworks,' they think it makes sense that every kid needs recess." Elizabeth Cushing, deputy director for strategy and development, added, "Those schools will demonstrate how play can impact learning and children's well-being. We are leveraging them to train other schools to do what we do. We are not satisfied with just direct service. We have a vision that every child in America's sixty thousand public schools will get to play every day. If we had enough money to serve every school directly with training, we would do it everywhere. But we don't."

The funding from the Robert Wood Johnson Foundation covers Sports4Kids' cost of operating in new schools, in declining amounts over three years to allow them time to find other money to cover this expense. The grant also added a $5 million line of credit to the $1.5 million the program had to cover expenses until schools paid their $23,500 fee each year. This expansion plan foresaw the most significant growth in the third and fourth years.

Sports4Kids ramped up its operations to manage this next expansion phase. It began planning one year in advance and had a recruitment team, personnel structure, and training in place so that the program was ready to run at the start of the new year. Again, Vialet sought out the principals who had buzz for being innovators, used the car GPS system, and dropped in on principals. The one-week demonstrations were again presented as a taste of what the program would be like.

"It's so difficult to explain the impact of this program unless you can actually see it and know how that whole demonstration week went for us," said Stevie Blakeley, principal at the Sacramento Elementary School in Portland. "Kids were beaming when they came off the playground. They would go back out and teach other kids, saying, 'Did you get to play this game? Let me show you how to do it.' I cannot tell you what a difference it made to have an extra person who really knew how to teach kids games and activities, keep them interested, and work with teachers. We saw a huge change in how our kids function on the playground and [in] their readiness to return to the classroom and learn."

—⟡— Economic Challenges and Sustainability

Sports4Kids—now Playworks—continues to generate effusive testimonials from children, parents, teachers, principals, and coaches themselves. Positive evaluations of its impact are starting to pile up. Kristen Madsen, a researcher at the University of California, Berkeley, Center for Weight and Health, examined findings of the annual California Healthy Kids Survey and concluded that "greater exposure to Playworks during elementary school was associated with greater meaningful participation in school, problem-solving skills, and increased physical activity."

Favorable news coverage continues to follow the program. Stories have appeared in local newspaper outlets, in prominent publications (such as *The Washington Post*), in television and radio features (such as NPR, the PBS *NewsHour*, and *ABC News*), and in a Portland, Oregon, television news feature. A New Orleans *Times-Picayune* headline proclaimed, "Peace recesses become child's play: Playground bullying at schools has decreased."

But there are doubters as well. *The New York Times* published an article in March 2010 citing people critical of the kind of approach used by Playworks as being overly regimented and not allowing children time to just relax. It quoted Romina Barros, an assistant clinical professor at New York's Albert Einstein College of Medicine who has published articles on the benefits of recess, as saying, "children still benefit most when they are let alone to daydream, solve problems, use their imagination to invent their own games, and 'be free to do what they choose to do.'"[8] One reader, commenting on the article online, wrote, "How sad. What about the kids who need some time to stare at clouds? What about the kids with lousy motor skills who now face another time when they feel like failures?"[9]

Most important, with money for schools so tight, nearly every extra expense, including Playworks, is carefully scrutinized. School districts with tight budgets must decide whether Playworks is so important that it shouldn't be touched or whether it is a program that, no matter how good it might be, must be forgone in times of economic hardship. Twenty-three thousand dollars is a lot of money for a strapped school district, and school superintendents, principals, and communities must decide whether Playworks is worth that investment. Some are answering that it is not and that they simply cannot afford the program.

Before the 2009–2010 school year, with the nation's economy in a tailspin, some retrenching had occurred. Playworks had operated in about a dozen middle and high schools in the Bay Area, and this was stopped. Nationally, the program expanded to about thirty fewer schools than planned in that year, also as a result of the bleak financial outlook. The program was beginning to miss growth targets, and with the largest expansion planned for years three and four (2011 and 2012), the program anticipated it would probably reach approximately 520 schools by 2012 (instead of 650).

During the 2009–2010 expansion push, the plan was for the organization to start up in New Orleans and St. Louis in the first year and then in Portland (Oregon), Newark, and Los Angeles in the second year. St. Louis was scrapped because of financial pressures and because schools there chose not to use the Title I money for the program, Vialet said. Playworks also aborted plans to serve Atlanta because the majority of schools there did not have recess and would not commit to instituting it.

A number of schools approached for this chapter either were unable to afford the program for the 2009–2010 school year or anticipated that they might have to drop Playworks the following year because of unusually grim school budget projections. Mildred Goss Elementary in San Jose reluctantly gave up the program in 2009–2010 when it had to make a difficult choice with shrinking resources between Playworks and another program that provided academic assistance during school. The school had been showcased in an NPR story about Sports4Kids, and the principal, teachers, parents, and kids had been wildly pleased about site coordinator Michelle Barron and the positive energy she brought to the school. "We talk about it a lot as a staff that so much has changed so quickly, how difficult it is to maintain Michelle's structure and order," said the principal, Brian Schmaedick. "In the two months since the year started, the environment on the playground has been slowly deteriorating." He said it was a "sad decision." In fact, the program was missed so much that the district decided to bring it back for the 2010–2011 school year and to expand it to other schools in the district as well. "We're making cuts in other areas to make it work," he said.

Even at Ohrenberger in Boston, the subject of the Harvard case study, the principal thought she might not be able to pay for Playworks in 2010–2011. "The program is great, but how do you sustain it during a fiscally tough time?" asked Eileen Nash, principal for Ohrenberger and Beethoven elementary schools, which both have Playworks. "We're all talking about it in Boston, how hard it is."

And Manzanita Community in Oakland expected it would probably give up Playworks in 2010 because the school district was requiring very steep budgetary cuts. For the principal Eyana Spencer, who had vowed that she would not run Manzanita without Playworks, this was a bitter pill. "It's unsettling because we're going into our fifth year with Playworks—how can we continue to make the gains we have if we cut this out?" she asked.

Playworks officials were sanguine about the schools' economic challenges, even as their biggest expansion targets yet were coming up in the next two years. Enough schools were continuing their commitment to the program, they said. Planning was in full swing in late 2009 to set up shop in six new cities for 2010–2011, and more schools were signing up for the program than ever, Vialet said. A major effort had been mounted to raise money, and it was going well, especially among individual donors, she said.

The biggest concern was California, where schools were more constrained because of the state's financial crisis. But Vialet was philosophical. "I am always worried, but am I more worried now? No," she said. "I knew when we got into this we were trying to do something extraordinarily difficult, so there is not a sudden awareness." The economy's historic decline may be giving Playworks just the push it needs to put the structure in place to weather these times, she said. "Not to be excessively Pollyanna about this, but trying to achieve scale and sustainability now might have been the best thing to happen to us because we have to do it in a solidly retail way, we have to build an infrastructure of support."

In recognition of the difficult economic situation, in 2009 Playworks made some critical changes. The city directors, who had largely focused on assuring the quality of the new programs in their city, became the executive directors and were charged primarily with raising funds locally from corporations and individuals donors. (Quality assurance was given to the area directors.) New hires were expected to have fundraising skills. It was the kind of work Vialet had excelled at, but she couldn't be everywhere, and the organization learned through experience that the leader of each city's program needed these fundraising skills, too. "The executive directors are the linchpins to each city's success," Elizabeth Cushing said. "They have to sell the program to everyone in the community and to funders. They have to be entrepreneurial and focus on building relationships and sales." The local advisory boards were revamped, too, taking a new form as boards of directors and receiving more responsibility for helping Playworks become financially strong.

The name of the program changed as well. "It was our experience that people assumed they knew what we did," Cushing said. "They were almost always wrong. They thought we did competitive sports like baseball or midnight basketball or that we did after-school sports. They never thought of four square or kickball or tag. That confusion was hard for us, particularly when we're trying to build new relationships to raise money." The program worked with a New York consulting firm, which conducted research with school principals, staff, and donors, and found that the name and logo did not readily communicate what the organization does. Many names were considered until Playworks was chosen and put in place in July 2009, along with the launch of a new Web site and logo.

Playworks also began a fee-supported technical assistance business, expecting to provide training to volunteer parents, teachers, and youth workers who could then bring its brand of play to hundreds of thousands more children. It began working with Head Start in New York City and in Stockton, California, schools.

Despite the economic situation, Playworks officials kept their eyes on the larger goal of building a movement for play that reaches all American schoolchildren, rich or poor. "We're tracking very well," said David Rothenberg, Playworks' executive director. "It's hard to keep people focused on a specific goal and reminding people that life is life. It's very likely our path will not mirror some line we had on a graph created in 2006 or 2007, but we continue to grow, and it's really impressive."

The organization has raised its profile significantly. It drew attention to itself as a leader in play in the nation's schools through its programs; media outreach; informative, attractively packaged materials; and an impressively designed, elaborate Web site. The Robert Wood Johnson Foundation report, *Recess Rules,* highlighted Playworks as it made the case for why recess is the ideal time for physical activity. The Foundation also produced a promotional video on the program that Playworks distributed. Playworks teamed up with the Cartoon Network, the National PTA, and others in a 2008 *Rescuing Recess* campaign to recruit volunteers to provide one million hours of physical activity and recess. In addition, Playworks won a Changemaker award in the Sport for a Better World competition sponsored by Nike and Ashoka.

In 2009, Playworks was invited to the White House three times, helping to supervise play in one of the visits during the annual Easter Egg Roll. Together with several other organizations, Vialet also worked with the White House Office of Social Innovation and Civic Participation to develop strategies for the First Lady to embrace in addressing the nation's physical inactivity crisis.

By the close of 2009, the organization that started out with two employees in 1996 in Berkeley had a staff of 264 employees and was making recess an enjoyable and healthy experience for seventy thousand low-income, inner-city children at 172 schools in ten cities. With the Foundation's second expansion grant ending in 2012, it is not yet clear whether the Robert Wood Johnson Foundation's support will continue. (Although, with AmeriCorps and other government funding contributing at least 15 percent of the expenses, schools paying 40 percent, and a major drive for fundraising reportedly succeeding, the program is likely to sustain itself at some level.) One thing remains unquestionable: this program of roshamboing, high-fiving, formerly unruly kids, inspiring coaches, and junior coaches who keep the playground safe and fun is meeting a need. "Playworks gives kids the opportunity to see that there is a different way to solve problems," said Ohrenberger's Eileen Nash, whose own school may be forced by economic reasons to drop the program. "When kids feel good about coming to school because they're not worried about conflicts, they're able to take pride in learning. This is one of the best things we can do for children."

Notes

1. Time Warner press release announcing the launch of the National Parent Teacher Association and Cartoon Network program. *Rescuing Recess*, March 13, 2006. http://www.timewarner.com/corp/newsroom/pr/0,20812,1172697,00.html.
2. National School Boards Association. "Time Out: Is Recess in Danger?" August 6, 2008. http://www.nsba.org/MainMenu/SchoolHealth/Search SchoolHealth/Time-Out.aspx.
3. Jarrett, O. S., Maxwell, D. M., Dickerson, C., Hoge, P., Davies, G., and Yetley, A. "The Impact of Recess on Classroom Behavior: Group Effects and Individual Differences." *Journal of Educational Research*, 1998, *92*, 121–126.
4. Ginsburg, K. R., Committee on Communications, and Committee on Psychosocial Aspects of Child and Family Health. "The Importance of Play in Promoting Healthy Child Development and Maintaining Strong Parent-Child Bonds." *Pediatrics*, 2007, *119*, 182–191.
5. Barros, R. M., Silver, E. J., and Stein, R. E. K. "School Recess and Group Classroom Behavior. *Pediatrics*, 2009, *123*, 431–436.
6. Harvard Family Research Project. "Evaluation Report: Case Study of the First Year of Sports4Kids at the Ohrenberger Elementary School in Boston, Massachusetts, 2006–2007 School Year." Harvard University Graduate School of Education. http://www.playworksusa.org/files/s4k_report_final.pdf.

7. Madsen, K., Crawford, P., and Campbell, E. "Improving Weight Status and Aerobic Fitness." *Sports4Kids Cumulative Report.* Dr. Robert C. and Veronica Atkins Center for Weight and Health, University of California at Berkeley, August 25, 2008.

8. Hu, W. "Forget Goofing Around: Recess Has a New Boss." *The New York Times,* March 14, 2010. http://community.nytimes.com/comments/www.nytimes.com/2010/03/15/education/15recess.html.

9. Comment 25 by "jwg" in ibid.

CHAPTER 4

Caring Across Communities

Will Bunch

Editors' Introduction

If one were to conduct a search for the most vulnerable population in the United States, children with mental health problems born to refugees or immigrants would surely be near the top. For starters, immigrants and their children are not generally welcome in the medical care system. If undocumented, they are pretty much precluded from getting care except in public hospitals, free clinics, and, to a limited extent, community health centers. They are more likely to live in poverty, be poorly educated, and lack health insurance coverage—with all the attendant consequences to health.

Then there is the question of obtaining mental health services. Despite laws and regulations requiring parity in coverage of mental and physical health services under employer-sponsored health plans, such parity does not in fact exist. Not to mention the stigma associated with mental illness, which would discourage many people from seeking services for themselves and their children.

Moreover, there are all of the cultural barriers, of which language is the most obvious and perhaps the easiest to resolve. In *The Spirit Catches You and You Fall Down,* Anne Fadiman writes poignantly about cultural misunderstanding between well-meaning American doctors and the equally well-meaning Hmong parents of an epileptic girl: "Many Hmong were overwhelmed. 'In America, we are blind because even though we have eyes, we cannot see. We are deaf because even though we have ears, we cannot hear.' Some newcomers wore pajamas as street clothes; poured water on electric stoves to extinguish them; lit charcoal fires in their living rooms; washed rice in their toilets [and] their clothes in swimming pools . . . . If the United States seemed incomprehensible to the Hmong, the Hmong seemed equally incomprehensible to the United States."[1]

In 2007, the Robert Wood Johnson Foundation launched a three-year program, Caring Across Communities, aimed at bringing school-connected mental health services to children of immigrants and refugees. Many refugees and their children have witnessed horrors unimaginable to most Americans. As a result, they suffer from post-traumatic stress disorder and are in great need of mental health services. In this chapter, Will Bunch, a prize–winning journalist with the *Philadelphia Daily News* and the author of the recent book, *The Backlash,* writes about Caring Across Communities. He describes the different approaches adopted by grantees in fifteen communities and examines lessons that have emerged from the program. With racial and ethnic minorities poised to become the majority of the population by 2042, programs such as Caring Across Communities will only increase in importance.

Note

1. Fadiman, A. *The Spirit Catches You and You Fall Down.* New York: Noonday Press, 1997, p. 188.

T here was no dramatic tipping point alerting public health officials in the United States of the need for specialized services for traumatized children of immigrants. However, by the late 1990s there was both an increase in, and a change in the nature of, new arrivals to America. In 2000, according to the Census Bureau, there were more than 31 million people in America who had been born somewhere else, a rise of 57 percent in just one decade, and many of those born elsewhere were schoolchildren.[1]

The mass migration took place despite domestic political currents hostile to immigration, especially toward those from Mexico and elsewhere in Latin America. On the southern border of the United States, children often arrived with the help of smugglers, surviving lethal heat and other brutal conditions. Meanwhile, a new surge of warfare across the Third World, especially in poverty-wracked Africa—frequently involving young people as victim or as child soldier—created new and previously unseen small pockets of immigration by legally protected refugees. With little cultural connection to America, they arrived in towns like Portland, Maine, and Fargo, North Dakota.

Studies show that one out of every five school children in America is now either the child of an immigrant or an immigrant him or her self—and the nature of the migration to this country is changing rapidly.[2] During the last three decades, the United States has accepted more refugees than the world's other developed nations combined, and increasingly these newcomers have been exposed to brutal modern warfare in Africa and elsewhere; thousands of children were killed, and many more were left psychologically scarred. Even economic refugees from Mexico and Central and South America faced new, lingering types of trauma as families were smuggled across the border in degrading conditions.

By the early 2000s, some experts were beginning to study the challenges these new arrivals faced in the area of mental health. Much of the evidence remained anecdotal. Foreign-born students who arrived under less stressful circumstances seemed to have mental health issues at about the same rate as American-born children; roughly one in ten kids receives medication or therapy.[3] But problems such as posttraumatic stress disorder (PTSD) appeared to be much more prevalent—closer to 20 percent—for those immigrants who experienced violence before arriving. School officials began to see the effects of PTSD in problems that ranged from rising individual disciplinary cases to a 25 percent high school dropout rate nationally for foreign-born pupils.[4] But no one had yet worked to develop a comprehensive strategy for tackling stress or related mental health issues among these children who seemed so clearly in need.

—⁓— Developing a Program to Address the Mental Health Needs of Refugees and Immigrants

Judith Stavisky, a former senior program officer for the Robert Wood Johnson Foundation who now heads the Philadelphia-based Friends of the Children, said that the Foundation began hearing reports in the early 2000s from grantees about difficulties they were facing in helping refugees and other immigrants make the transition to life in America. In 2003, she and Foundation program officer Wendy Yallowitz traveled the country to visit agencies on the front lines working with such refugees.

Stavisky said she was especially moved by the struggles of newcomers she met on a trip to Omaha, where many Sudanese, Somali, Burmese, Latino, and other refugees had come to work in the local meatpacking industry. She was also handed a book by a well-known local therapist, Mary Pipher, called *The Middle of Everywhere: Helping Refugees Enter the American Community,* which depicted in great and occasionally almost comic detail the problems that Sudanese and other refugees encountered in Nebraska. It described some of their underlying traumas and called for "cultural brokers" who would work full time with refugees—as a practical nurse might—to help them adjust. The site visits and the timely book convinced Stavisky and her colleagues at the Foundation to devise a program to address the mental health needs of these immigrants.

"Some of these children had seen unthinkable things—they had seen torture, for example, and they had lived in these camps, or they had been homeless," Stavisky said. "Then they come to school in America—and they're not even wearing the right clothes. So a lot of this was: How do we overcome this, and make sure that this accumulation of hurt and losses that they have is recognized?"

Julia Graham Lear, the former director of and now senior advisor to the Center for Health and Health Care in Schools at George Washington University, who has worked with the Foundation on child health issues for more than two decades, was also intrigued by what the research was showing and by how little Americans knew about the issues that refugees encountered. Lear pointed to the little-understood ways that immigrating to America frequently ripped apart families—especially for those coming from war-torn Africa. "Here's the deal—you get a visa to the United States when you're in the refugee camp through a lottery system, but the child is not in the lottery, it's the adult," Lear explained. "But when an adult was tapped for resettlement in the United States, she often would take as many children as she could, regardless of whether or not they were her own biological kids—a situation that might make kids physically safer but could be damaging psychologically."

A new initiative seemed a logical step for the Foundation, which had recently created its Vulnerable Populations portfolio to address the areas in American life where health problems were exacerbated by social factors such as poverty, violence, and substandard living conditions. Yallowitz said a plan was created to reach immigrant children through the most obvious point of contact, the public schools. "We wanted to narrow it down to where we could make the biggest impact, and schools were where they were spending the majority of their time," Yallowitz said.

The Foundation and Lear had already worked to establish the very first school-based health centers, primarily in underserved communities. The efforts began in the early 1970s with a pilot program, the School Health Services program, that placed nurse practitioners in elementary schools in four states; in 1986, the Foundation launched a more ambitious, seven-year nationwide program called the School-Based Adolescent Health Care program, which helped create a template for treatment that today is used in many of the nearly two thousand such school-based health centers in the United States. To build its mental health effort for refugees, the Foundation turned to Lear.

In 2006, the Foundation announced a first-of-its-kind initiative, Caring Across Communities, to target immigrant and refugee populations in fifteen communities. The goal was to develop different models and a variety of approaches—sharing information during the three-year life of the program; at the end of the thirty-six months, the Foundation could apply the knowledge developed through the pilot program to promulgate best practices and to develop working programs in immigrant communities across the United States.

The Foundation allocated $7 million over three years for the Caring Across Communities program and selected Lear's Center for Health and Health Care in Schools to administer it. Each of the fifteen sites would receive up to $100,000 a year over the three years. The roster of projects unveiled in March 2007 showcased a variety of approaches in locations ranging from the sun-baked, overwhelmingly Latino Imperial County, California, on the Mexican border, to the northern climes of Fargo, North Dakota—a destination for a surprising number of refugees from an array of nations.

The common thread throughout this variety of programs was the school. "That was because most refugee parents coming to

America in pursuit of a better life for children understood the importance of a good education," Olga Acosta Price, director of the Center for Health and Health Care in Schools, said. "Thus parents would be more willing to work with a program with a focus on mental health if it were framed and explained as a way to keep kids in school and help them to achieve."

—ᨳ— A Variety of Approaches: Caring Across Communities in Practice

After the first two years of the Caring Across Communities program—a period of trial and error but also of encouraging stories—many of the fifteen programs had already become established fixtures in the communities they served. Here is the in-depth story of site visits to two of the local sites.

Boston, Massachusetts

At 10:45 on a Tuesday morning, half a dozen boys from the seventh and eighth grades slowly file down a hallway inside Boston's Lilla G. Frederick Pilot Middle School, their heels clicking on the glossy floor of their ultra-modern, Wi-Fi–enabled high-tech haven located amid the peeling multifamily homes of the city's rugged Dorchester section. The boys have a lot in common and are wiry, dark-skinned, and bantering in accents of their homeland, Somalia. They file into a conference room, where for the next fifty minutes they'll take a break from online algebra lessons and do something normally quite unremarkable for young teenagers—compete against each other or with two adults in board games like tic-tac-toe-inspired Connect 4 or Jenga, the block-stacking game.

The Somali-born boys are mostly quiet as they play, the squeaking of their chairs across the floor interrupted only by the collapse of a towering Jenga stack, accompanied by a "Ya!" or a self-satisfied declaration of victory. "Piece of cake, I win!" declares one of the boys after besting one of his friends at Connect 4, and there are good-natured smiles and murmurs around a big table. One of the two adult leaders, Saida Abdi, who is herself a native of Somalia, reminds the young immigrants about the importance of taking deep breaths to relax. At the end of the hour, she turns to Amanda Nisewaner—also a social worker in the novel refugee aid program called Project SHIFA (for Supporting the Health of Immigrant Families and Adolescents; *shifa* means "healing" in Arabic)—and declares, "I am very proud of them, Amanda. They played for a long time, and they did it by themselves."

When Abdi and other social workers started working with Boston's Somali refugee community several years ago, such a placid hour of group play would have been impossible: The boys were prone to fights over minor slights, and several even found it difficult to sit still for such a long period. Their difficulties in adjusting to life in an American middle school should not have been a surprise; most of the youth were just a couple of years removed from a grim existence in Kenyan-based refugee camps for the thousands displaced by years of brutal warfare in their neighboring failed state on the Horn of Africa, and some had already seen brutal murders or abandoned corpses in the streets or felt the fear of a hasty flight at the point of a rifle. Resettlement in the United States was a step toward a better life, but in addition to the traditional burdens of learning a new language and culture, many of these young refugees from war had to also overcome PTSD, along with other mental-health issues.

It's a vexing problem to the educators, social workers, and mental health professionals who are aware of it. But Project SHIFA—led by Children's Hospital Boston, working closely with members of the local Somali community as well as schools and Somali community agencies, and funded by the Robert Wood Johnson Foundation—has made considerable headway in just a couple of years. Its efforts have been increasingly focused on raising awareness among parents, religious leaders, and other key figures in Boston's still-growing

Somali community about the importance of mental health, while breaking down considerable cultural stigmas surrounding mental health issues.

Since it was launched, in 2007, Project SHIFA has worked with dozens of Somali teens and pre-teens and their families in informal settings like the weekly discussion and play group at the Dorchester school; officials boast a hundred percent success rate in engaging once-reluctant parents to seek help when more intensive therapy is needed. Heidi Ellis, a clinical psychologist at Children's Hospital and associate director of its Center for Refugee Trauma and Resilience, who launched the project to address the growing Somali caseload, said that a key was cutting through taboos. "The idea of a kid having some problems or being a little stressed or distressed about something—most families would look at that and say, 'Don't call my child crazy,'" she said.

Ellis said the tide began to turn after a parent outreach director, Somali-born Naima Agalab, held a Ramadan tea for forty refugee mothers and convinced them that it was better to join the system of counseling in American schools than to resist it. "'This is real, this is happening,'" she recounted Agalab telling the immigrants, "'and instead of just denying it and wishing that kids weren't going to mental health professionals, we need to get involved in it—so that we are confident that the services that are happening can really help our kids and not hurt them.'"

These struggles are hardly isolated to refugees from Somalia or Boston. In many ways, Project SHIFA—working amid a growing Somali community of about eight thousand people—is typical of the Caring Across Communities grantees.

The idea was hatched several years ago when a couple of cases from the Boston school district involving Somalis with disciplinary problems were referred to Ellis, who was then working through an immigrant-based psychology clinic at Boston Medical Center. Ellis said she quickly realized that these young refugees were coping with enormous trauma—not just from their war-torn past but now from adjusting to life in some of Boston's rougher neighborhoods and public schools. In addition, the hurdles in connecting these refugees with the proper treatment were quite high, indeed. Although most of the children were quick to pick up English, their parents often didn't speak the language, were unfamiliar with how things worked in an American school, and were reluctant to agree to the kind of intense aid that some of the children clearly required.

What's more, the classroom teachers frequently didn't have the time (or even the interest) to explore the deeper reasons for a student's acting out in the classroom. There were few Somali teachers in the entire Boston school system, and not one mental health professional that Ellis could find in the entire state of Massachusetts who could speak the Somali language or had any familiarity with the distinctive culture of the East African nation. It quickly became clear that a huge problem would be simply winning acceptance for Western ideas about mental health care.

Several years later, half a dozen or so mothers of Somali-born Boston school students are sitting around a windowless conference room inside the city's Refugee and Immigrant Assistance Center, an old brewery building in the city's Jamaica Plain neighborhood. Dressed in blindingly bright *guntiinos* (full-length dresses), in head scarves, and munching on pastries as they speak in their native Somali tongue, the women are all members of a parent advisory board that has proved critical in helping Ellis and her small team of social workers gain acceptance and understanding.

"In our country, we do not have these terms like bipolar or manic-depressive," says one of the women through a translator, smiling at how much she had learned about the subject of mental health in just a couple of years. "In our country, you are not 'crazy' unless you are running around in the street with no clothes on!" The others in the group of refugee moms laugh heartily. The fact that the Boston-based Somalis can joke about such once-taboo topics is a sign of how far Project SHIFA has been able to reach into the community in just a couple of years.

How did this happen? Ellis and her growing team of psychologist colleagues and social workers broadened their strategy to go well beyond just therapy sessions for the most troubled kids: They added Somali natives like Abdi, who brought credibility and also did extensive outreach work to educate schoolteachers about the unique problems of refugee children; then they met with parents and with Islamic religious leaders in the immigrant community to boost awareness. In a sense, Project SHIFA created its own nomenclature as the social workers learned ways to get parents and kids to trust in its work initially without even using the phrase *mental health* or related terms, for fear of scaring would-be clients away. Now its team holds weekly meetings on the Children's Hospital campus to develop treatment strategies for Somali teens who once would have been lost deep in the system.

On a Monday morning, roughly ten professionals sit around a large table to discuss the progress of some of their more intensely managed cases—allowing both the author and a visiting film crew to observe as long as names of the individual students are withheld. In addition to staff psychologists, the team includes Abdi, who has often visited the families in their homes, as well as Nisewaner, who spends a good portion of her time at the middle school in Dorchester when she is not studying toward her social work degree at Boston University through a Project SHIFA–related program. (Since this scene took place, Nisewaner completed her studies and was hired by the project.) Nisewaner spoke at length about a boy who was born in one of the Somali refugee camps in neighboring Kenya, the oldest of several siblings, who has had a tough time in school with fights and other temper flare-ups. As the oldest child, and because of the violence and squalor he witnessed in the camp, Nisewaner speculated, the student seemed constantly worried about protecting his mother.

"He felt like he should be at home," Nisewaner said, explaining why he didn't find pleasure in playing soccer with some of the other Somali boys after school. "He felt like he was too old to be out playing." She described bumpy progress, but the young social worker said she believed that counseling had helped the boy avoid what could have been a violent confrontation with a group of kids in the neighborhood. The staff around the table agreed that the boy was not currently in need of crisis-level intervention, although Ellis asked, "'Is there any way to get the school to give him some positive feedback?'"

The case sums up much of what educators, psychologists, and social workers from the sunny Los Angeles barrio to foggy Portland, Maine, have discovered during the three years of the Caring Across Communities experiment: regardless of culture, advocates for treatment can break down the barriers of social traditions and language and make a difference in the lives of at least some families—but the work is difficult and time-consuming. With the three-year pilot ending in 2010, leaders of most of the fifteen Caring Across Communities projects were turning their attention toward the problem of finding a sustainable funding base in a rough economy, so that more kids like this struggling Somali boy in Dorchester could be helped in the future.

Bucks County, Pennsylvania

George Wion speaks slowly, in raspy, lilting tones of his native Liberia, frequently burying his bald head into his hands when asked about his family's life in the war-torn African nation or about his son—also named George—and some of the awful things that George Jr. and his siblings witnessed in Liberia, where civil war between 1999 and 2003 killed an estimated two hundred thousand people. Wion and his family, including three kids, immigrated to the United States in July 2005, but their new life in the working-class suburbs just north of Philadelphia also brought new problems.

When the younger George Wion was in seventh grade at the Franklin D. Roosevelt Middle School in Bristol Township,

Pennsylvania, he fell in with some kids involved in gang activity. "He was getting along, but the problem was there were some kids here that used to take him along to all kinds of places," the father said. "He was getting friendly with some bad boys, and every time he comes to school sometimes he didn't come home, and when he was home sometimes they would come over very late."

The older George Wion was separated from his wife and wasn't around much himself. He worked long hours at a residential youth home in a different community in suburban Bucks County. But partly on the recommendation of a Liberian Christian minister who is well-known among Bristol Township's small, tight-knit refugee community, the senior Wion gave his permission for his son to work with a school-based Caring Across Communities project run by the Family Services Association of Bucks County. The program sought to go beyond traditional therapy, not only with more intensive one-on-one counseling in the schools but also through home visits, family counseling, and other forms of community outreach. In young George's case, working with a social worker, Allison Taite-Tarver, based at the middle school, and with a school psychologist helped him improve both his grades and his self-esteem. Taite-Tarver made frequent visits to the family's home for additional counseling and even visited their church; she and a colleague then worked with them to prepare an application to transfer to a Christian boarding school in Indiana, a long way from urban gang activity. The application was successful.

Taite-Tarver concedes that in helping young George Wion adjust to—and then leave—Bucks County, the program barely scratched the surface of the teen's experiences in Liberia, where the family frequently moved around at the barrel of a gun. In an interview, the father filled in some of the blanks. "We were going from place to place, looking for food for the kids, and we had to go through all kinds of stuff," he said. "They would kill people, and they would be lying there dead in the street. But the kids were still little . . . ."

Ironically, the now famous phrase that "it takes a village to raise a child" is an African proverb, but it is here in Bucks County that the phrase came to life for George Wion Jr. and also for some of the other adolescent children among the estimated two hundred or so Liberians who resettled in Bucks County.

That's because the program in Bucks County came together through the efforts of a diverse team, including an enthusiastic principal at the FDR Middle School eager for outside help with its new Liberian students and other nontraditional immigrants. She was aided by staff members at the county mental health agency and at the Family Service Association, a nonprofit mental health and counseling agency. A suburban county such as Pennsylvania's Bucks has more resources than some cash-strapped locales, but officials still had a hard time delivering social services to the small number of Liberians who began trickling in roughly a decade ago, at the height of the civil war. Even though Liberians arrived speaking English, removing one barrier, officials said, early relief efforts by Catholic Social Services faltered. County mental health services were geared to interventions that could be billed to the federal Medicaid program. They did not provide for the more broadly based family and school outreach envisioned by the Caring Across Communities grant—especially the community work, home visits, and family therapy efforts that were not covered by insurance—and the services that were available were difficult to access, especially by people who were working.

The program's most enthusiastic booster is the school's principal, Ruth Geissel, who began in 2006 and saw a few Liberian-born students involved in an alarming number of fights, especially with a much larger and entrenched group of African Americans. "The students coming in were used to fighting," Geissel said, referring to Liberian teens who had spent their formative years in a refugee camp. "So it was much easier for them to fight than to work things out." Officials with the refugee-counseling partnership that came together in Bucks County agree that the interest that Geissel and other school officials showed in a full-time social worker inside the school and in outreach to the community on the outside (in some other locales there has been resistance to these kind of programs) has been critical to the success of the effort; the principal even donated her own conference room so Taite-Tarver could work with students.

Another beneficial move was hiring a Liberian native named Abraham Kamara Jr., who first came to the United States in the 1970s with his single mother and was educated in American schools. Kamara has kept one foot planted in Liberian culture; he had already been working closely with the refugee community in Bucks County as a caseworker for Planned Parenthood when he was brought on to help the Family Service Association promote its efforts.

"I went into the churches, because you have to do it outside the box," Kamara said. In many ways, he has been the kind of cultural broker the Nebraska writer Pipher had envisioned. In his part-time role, he not only went to religious services and soccer games but spent considerable time on aid that was tangential to mental health, such as housing, medical referrals, immigration-law problems, and connecting Liberians with food pantries. "You have to come at them with respect—you have to engage in a conversation [about] being in this country and the opportunities that are given here, compared to being in Liberia," said Kamara, who splits his time between the middle school and home and church visits. He said he understood the complexities of Liberian family life, including male dominance in household affairs, and often swept-under-the-rug problems caused by children coming to America with adults who are not their biological parents. Having an educated Liberian-American to talk to "just raises their self-esteem, makes them feel good about themselves," Kamara said.

—⚌— Diverse Approaches from Coast to Coast

Some communities used Robert Wood Johnson Foundation funding to develop a strategy different than those employed in Boston and Bucks County, where programs targeted a specific refugee group. In Portland, Maine, school officials found that their midsized New England city (population sixty-five thousand) was flooded with new arrivals from all over the globe—Cambodia, Somalia, Serbia, Vietnam, and Latin America, among other places—and that the existing network of social services was ill-equipped to meet refugees' needs. About sixteen hundred of the seven thousand public school students in Portland were taking English as a second language (ESL) classes.

Grace Valenzuela, who directs the Portland Caring Across Communities project and is also assistant for multicultural affairs to the schools superintendent, said that "we were in silos"—with too little to bridge steep walls between the teachers, the guidance counselors, the social workers who worked with local immigrant groups, and the public mental health staffers who could treat the most trauma-stricken students. Although the resources to work with refugees with PTSD were largely in place, the missing pieces of the puzzle in Portland were largely twofold: (1) upgrading the cultural competence of the key players within the schools and social services, and (2) building trust with the immigrant parents to convince them to avail themselves of these services.

At the launch of the Portland program, its organizers worked with so-called consultants—community members who might receive gift certificates or other minimal compensation for their efforts—to understand what the needs of the city's different immigrant communities were. From that, a series of roughly thirty workshops for Portland's professionals were held over the next three years on topics ranging from resettlement issues and immigration law to working with interpreters and notions of family and kinship. In addition to the knowledge that was shared, these sessions led to better communication between the once- isolated agencies. There were even one-on-one sessions between social workers and various healers within the refugee communities—all with the goal of improving cultural competence.

"We've learned that we have to shift the paradigm for healing as it exists—that we're in a box and it's been arbitrarily created for us by a system that really doesn't do the work: they do things like insurance coverage," said Lisa Belanger, the city of Portland's family health program manager. She said the goal of the program in Portland and many of the other projects in Caring Across Communities was nothing less than "a revolution" in health care for refugees, centered less on top-down mandates about coverage and American notions of mental health best practices and more on the bottom-up cultural needs and related issues surrounding migrants. Growth of the Caring Across Communities program was analogous to the hospice movement, which arose from the failure of the health care and insurance industries to develop a system of care for the dying much as schools and some government agencies were oblivious to mental health problems among refugees. In three years, project leaders said the Portland program was able to offer counseling services to 153 students, often working closely with their families.

Despite obstacles, the program in Maine had an advantage that was not shared by some of the other Caring Across Communities projects. The Maine program had a supportive political climate, including many non-immigrant parents who cherished the diversity the public schools in Maine had to offer. But that was not the case in every locale where the Caring Across Communities projects operated. The 2000s were defined in much of the United States by a political climate of increasing resentment from native-born American citizens toward immigrants who did not speak English or who lacked proper documentation, or both. In search of a decent wage, many refugees flooded rural Sunbelt communities that were not used to handling students from non-English-speaking homes, let alone to offering special services for trauma. Political resentment flourished in these communities.

Chatham County, North Carolina, a rural area south of the university town of Chapel Hill, is such a place; its town of Siler City was considered a model for television's Mayberry, the iconic fictional small southern town depicted on *The Andy Griffith Show* in the 1960s. Today, roughly half of this small town is made up of immigrants, mostly Spanish-speaking families from Mexico or Central America who were lured by work in a chicken processing plant that closed in 2008. The influx has not always been welcome; the notorious ex-Klan leader David Duke even held a rally in Siler City where he asked several hundred people, "To get a few chickens plucked—is it worth losing your heritage?"

In the county schools, officials report that about fifteen hundred of the seven thousand students are either Hispanic immigrants or the children of immigrants. As with refugee children from war zones, preliminary studies indicate high rates of mental health problems. Some 59 percent of the immigrant children are suffering from symptoms of anxiety, about one-third are dealing with PTSD, and 9 percent have had thoughts of suicide—and yet rates of treatment are appallingly low. When Caring Across Communities was launched in 2007, Mimi Chapman, an associate professor in the School of Social Work at the University of North Carolina, seized the opportunity to partner with the county school system and with El Futuro, a program that aggressively promotes and offers mental health programs for local immigrants. The new partnership would be named Creating Confianza.

"A lot of these kids have problems because they were exposed to violence or to other traumatic life experiences," said Chapman. She said that many of the Latino immigrant children experienced harrowing journeys from Mexico or elsewhere in Latin America with their parents who were in search of work. "I don't think their teachers realize what they went through," she said. "They have no idea that they saw people dying in the desert, or that they were kept alive on boxes of rice."

Unlike some of its northern counterparts in the Caring Across Communities network, the district in Chatham County did not have a history of offering school-based mental health services to students. In launching Creating Confianza for the immigrant student population, Chapman and her partners were forced to create that foundation from scratch, working with parents and others to create a mental health advisory board. Although a cornerstone of the program was hiring a full-time, Spanish-speaking social worker—called a school-family liaison—based in the county's middle and high schools, Creating Confianza learned that some of its most successful work was simply raising the awareness level of teachers about some of the issues their new students faced as immigrants. In one typical case, the liaison interceded on behalf of a Mexican-born, Spanish-speaking new arrival at his middle school who was uncommunicative and sometimes failed to show up at all. The liaison learned that the youth had developed poor attendance habits in Mexico, where he was often unable to attend his school because of local flooding. Simply learning the student's troubled background and explaining his story to his teachers, Chapman reported, created a climate of improved compassion.

Creating Confianza workers found the bulk of their work involved achieving what it called "climate change" in the Chatham schools—for example, making sure a simultaneous translation machine was hooked up and working for parent-teacher meetings; the expensive device had been sitting idle, remarkably, for six years. Chapman and her team also went to great lengths to design two-hour sessions for parents. To encourage attendance, dinner and childcare were provided. At these sessions, the adults were asked to react to certain vignettes, told in such a way as to de-emphasize that the cases were mental health problems. Creating Confianza later reported that nine families asked El Futuro for counseling after these meetings. Chapman said that "ninety-five percent of the parents tell us, 'Yes, these problems are important—but I wouldn't know where to go for help.' Only three percent have sought mental health services. That's a good indication that we need parents who are willing to participate."

Rural Imperial County, California, which borders Mexico and Arizona, lies to the east of the San Diego metropolitan area. The mostly agricultural county's population is roughly 75 percent Hispanic, mixing Mexican-American families who have been there for three or four generations with newly arrived immigrant families. Nearly a third of the county's current population was born in Mexico. Here, Caring Across Communities financed a project that grew out of a longstanding project, Proyecto Puentes (the Bridges Project), which targeted mental health issues for students in two communities: Calexico, just across the border from the sprawling city of Mexicali, and Heber, an unincorporated community nearby with high poverty levels.

George Miranda, the longtime administrator of family services and student well-being in Imperial County, said social workers in the Bridges Project learned that some families who had been on the U.S. side of the border for a number of years continued to struggle with acculturation, language issues, and poverty. The Robert Wood Johnson Foundation grant allowed Proyecto Puentes to hire two bilingual *promotoras,* who worked with school staff, held weekly sessions with small groups of students in two junior high schools, and launched outreach efforts to parents. "They know the culture, they've grown up in the Valley, and they make personal contact with follow-up visits to the homes," Miranda said of the *promotoras.* "They [have] also mastered the art of avoiding cultural stigmas by discussing mental health issues with families in terms of everyday stress."

By the end of the second full year, more than three hundred students at the two schools had been connected to outside support services, and some thirty-four of these—kids who otherwise most likely would have fallen through the cracks—had received mental health services. "You need a lot of people to just get out there and talk to them and connect with them," Miranda said. Still, as the Caring Across Communities funding neared its end, Miranda seemed overwhelmed at trying to tackle these issues with only two full-time people. "It's not a lot of resources, really—we need more support," Miranda said.

—〜— Taking Stock

Miranda's comments summed up the broader mood of those who had participated in Caring Across Communities as the three-year funding window was about to shut. There was optimism that the projects could make a difference for immigrant students and their families, tempered by the realization that models for a successful program are expensive, and options for future funding are limited.

Yet despite the limited time frame of the Caring Across Communities program and the uncertain funding prospects, those involved with Caring Across Communities said that in three years these pilot projects had accumulated a number of lessons to offer to others contemplating programs to improve mental health for immigrant and refugee children and their families. These lessons include the following:

1. *Cultural competence is key.* Many of the individual Caring Across Communities projects reported that their greatest progress came when they were able to identify and hire individuals or mental health professionals who came from the same country or ethnic background as the refugee population they were trying to serve. Most leaders said that these cultural brokers—who not only spoke the language but also understood taboos and culturally based selling points for wary refugee families—were the missing link that led to surprisingly high rates of parental participation.

Lear, the founder of the Center for Health and Health Care in Schools, said that working with community groups or social workers from the same culture as the refugees was important because immigrants might have been scared away by an imposing expert-heavy, mental health–only oriented approach. "As a culture, America really values expertise—and that is not a bad thing," Lear said. "However, if the expertise is not going to be a source of enlightenment, it can be a barrier."

2. *The notion of building programs around the schools is a good one.* The public schools are clearly a focal point for immigrant and refugee families; that is especially true for programs such as the Caring Across Communities efforts in California and North Carolina, which targeted students born in Mexico or Central America where many parents lacked documentation and had few other contact points with official institutions. Likewise, many refugees—both political and economic—have placed many of their hopes for life in the United States on the education of their children, which is why school achievement is more likely to be a trigger for accepting aid, especially mental health counseling. "If you don't have the commitment from the schools, then the program doesn't work," said Yallowitz, the program officer with the Robert Wood Johnson Foundation.

3. *Effective programs involve a wide partnership of school, community, and governmental groups.* The staff members who planned and organized the Caring Across Communities program said they felt vindicated in their original idea of a partnership model that connected existing community groups with school and mental health professionals. In communities with sophisticated social services infrastructures—such as those in Portland, Maine, and Boston—project organizers saw that all the key elements were in place. However, before the Caring Across Communities involvement, organizers were not communicating with one another. In more isolated or more poverty-stricken areas, the challenge instead was to take an existing asset—the in-school social services that already existed in Imperial County, California, for example—and use that as a base for building a new project.

4. *Parents must become stakeholders in the program.* Many of the programs put considerable resources into outreach programs aimed not only at telling families about the existence of the project but also convincing them of its merits. One of the more ambitious efforts was created by the Caring Across Communities program in San Jose, California and was named Project Tam An. Project Tam An was an Asian American Recovery Services program that targeted Vietnamese refugees. The project secured a fifteen-minute weekly slot on a community radio show and ran ads in the ethnic

newspaper for the region's Vietnamese. The radio show featured conversations with parents and teens (or with mental health professionals) and was aimed at combating the notion among parents that problems like PTSD were not treatable but were simply the result of "bad karma." Many of the Caring Across Communities projects also invested considerable resources in high-quality brochures or in sponsoring community breakfasts, all aimed at raising parent awareness and fighting stigmas and other fears.

Some of the directors of the fifteen individual Caring Across Communities projects came to learn that parents—perhaps intimidated by the American school systems—didn't think it was their role to get involved in such matters at first, but responded positively when they were sought out. "These refugee parents resettled here for their children," said Kristen Huffman-Gottschling of the Caring Across Communities project called World Relief-Chicago, which works with a polyglot of immigrant and refugee groups. "They [parents] are fully invested in their children's future."

To reach those parents, however, it was critical for the project leaders to forge close working relationships with already existing social service agencies that had strong roots and had built trust within a particular immigrant community; trusted agency staff could serve as cultural guides and interpreters.

As the program began winding down in late 2009, the Robert Wood Johnson Foundation hired an evaluator, Clea McNeely, assistant professor in the department of public health at the University of Tennessee and an expert in adolescent mental health issues, to study five Caring Across Communities projects in depth to identify lessons that could guide similar programs in the future. Speaking in general terms about the programs, before her findings were published in 2010, McNeely noted that Caring Across Communities projects often found they had to deal with other barriers of poverty, cultural divides, and the day-to-day needs of employment or food before they could even reach the point where intensive mental health treatment made sense.

McNeely said that the stronger projects she witnessed were moving away from a narrow focus on placing some refugee and immigrant kids into mental health counseling programs and were instead taking a more holistic approach to the range of problems that refugees face. "What is stress?" McNeely asked. "It's moving to a neighborhood where's there is crime and no jobs, where you are unable to get a driver's license." She joined program officials in noting that refugee families experience certain kinds of problems not typically addressed by traditional American treatment models, including the language barriers that often cause teens to assume adult roles in the family as well as a frequently voiced fear by parents that an angry child could report them for abuse and they could lose custody as a result.

McNeely said she would advise projects not to adhere too closely to what she called "the trauma model" of seeking to cull the most serious cases of PTSD or other severe mental health crises, but to instead move toward offering a much more broadly based set of services.

McNeely also noted that programs such as Caring Across Communities placed a heavy load on teachers, whose workday was already full. "The teachers need to teach," she said, "and they're being asked to do a lot more"—while often lacking both resources and the time to communicate with project staff members about individual students. "The stronger programs actually took the burden off the teachers' shoulders," McNeely continued. "The teachers loved it, and it helped them deal with problems that they were unequipped to handle or didn't have time for."

Indeed, McNeely said her evaluation research found that the Caring Across Communities projects were fighting what she believed to be an uphill battle against inadequate support for resettled refugees in general: the federal law on assistance for refugees, which had not been updated since 1980, was finally amended in 2009. McNeely notes that refugees receive only $1,100, which must last them for four months and out of which they typically have to pay rent, purchase food and transportation, buy clothes, and take care of their basic necessities. Immigrants, McNeely noted, often face economic challenges even more severe than those faced by refugees.

The annual fall gathering of the Caring Across Communities partners held in Washington, D.C., in the fall of 2009 centered on what was now the most critical issue: program sustainability.

At that conference, there was considerable sharing of information about which services could be billed for reimbursement by the Medicaid program, which typically covers resettled refugees and identifies regional grant makers who might consider supporting the more broadly based immigrant services. Despite the lingering effects of the American economic slowdown and disappointment about having lost support from the Robert Wood Johnson Foundation, many of the Caring Across Communities program leaders felt that the breakthroughs they had seen in just three years should bring new attention and sources of support—especially when so much more remains to be learned about refugees and their mental health issues.

The program's leaders take pride in the individual children they have helped, including a case that Lear witnessed on a visit to Boston, where a Somali teen in the middle school was observed by teachers as isolated, angry, and acting out. "It turned out," Lear recalled, "that the rumor had gone around the school that this boy was a boy soldier. The teachers were able to sit down with both the refugee community and with people who know something about treatment, and ask, 'How do we deal with a situation like this?'" It was another case that showed that, regardless of whether the setting is Africa or America, quite often it can still take a village to save a child.

Notes

1. U. S. Census Bureau. "The Foreign-Born Population, 2000: Census 2000 Brief." December 2003. http:www.census.gov/prod/2003pubs/c2kbr-34.pdf.

2. Suárez-Orozco, C., and Suárez-Orozco, M. *Children of Immigration.* Cambridge, Mass.: Harvard University Press, 2001. http://www.hepg .org/her/booknote/112.

3. Simpson, G. A., Cohen, R. A., Pastor, P. N., and Reuben, C. A. "U.S. Children 4–17 Years of Age Who Received Services for Emotional or Behavioral Difficulties. Preliminary Data from the 2005 National Health Interview Survey." CDC National Center for Health Statistics, 2006. http://www.cdc.gov/nchs/data/hestat/children2005/children2005.htm.

4. Fry, R. "The Higher Drop-Out Rate of Foreign-Born Teens." Pew Hispanic Center, November 1, 2005. http://pewhispanic.org/reports/report.php? ReportID=55.

CHAPTER 5

The United Teen Equality Center in Lowell, Massachusetts

Digby Diehl

Editors' Introduction

Some of the Robert Wood Johnson Foundation's most interesting grantees and programs have come from the Robert Wood Johnson Foundation Local Funding Partnerships program or, as it was called in the past, the Local Initiative Funding Partners program. Through this program, local foundations identify innovative health or health care programs that touch the lives of individuals in the community and nominate them for joint funding with the Robert Wood Johnson Foundation. This mechanism has allowed the Foundation to support a diverse group of programs, such as those that provide substance abuse treatment for Lakota Sioux living in South Dakota,[1] prenatal care for pregnant homeless women in San Francisco,[2] basic dental services for Alaskans living in remote areas,[3] and vaccinations for older Americans going to vote.[4]

Through the Local Funding Partnerships program, the Foundation has supported programs to stop gang violence in inner cities. In volume VIII of the *Anthology,* Digby Diehl, a regular contributor to the *Anthology* series whose most recent book collaboration, *Patti Lupone: A Memior*, appeared in 2010, wrote about the Chicago Project for Violence Prevention, a program that attempts to curb gang violence in Chicago by treating it as analogous to a public health problem.[5] In this chapter, Diehl examines another approach to stemming gang violence, this one taken by the United Teen Equality Center in Lowell, Massachusetts. The program uses *streetworkers,* some of whom were former gang members themselves, to stop outbreaks of gang violence and help gang members get an education, locate employment training opportunities, and find jobs.

As is the case with many of the programs supported by Local Funding Partnerships, this program was the brainchild of a farsighted individual who had a vision of how life in the community could be made better, pursued the vision, and was able to attract foundation support to develop and nurture it. The chapter offers both a case study of an innovative program and a portrayal of the people who make this program a reality.

Notes

1. Diehl, D. "The Catholic Social Services Outreach Project." *To Improve Health and Health Care, Vol. XII: The Robert Wood Johnson Foundation Anthology.* San Francisco: Jossey-Bass, 2009.
2. Diehl, D. "The Homeless Prenatal Program." *To Improve Health and Health Care, Vol. VII: The Robert Wood Johnson Foundation Anthology.* San Francisco: Jossey-Bass, 2004.
3. See Chapter 6.
4. Brodeur, P. "SPARC-Sickness Prevention Achieved Through Regional Collaboration." *To Improve Health and Health Care, Vol. X: The Robert Wood Johnson Foundation Anthology.* San Francisco: Jossey-Bass, 2006.
5. Digby D. "The Chicago Project for Violence Prevention." *To Improve Health and Health Care, Vol. VIII: The Robert Wood Johnson Foundation Anthology.* San Francisco: Jossey-Bass, 2000.

—∿— **W**hen the dismissal bell rings at 2:30 P.M. every weekday afternoon, a river of teenagers flows out the doors of Lowell High School, down the steps, and onto city sidewalks. With an enrollment of more than four thousand students, Lowell is the second-largest high school in Massachusetts.

There is a great deal of history in Lowell. In the early nineteenth century, it was the first hot spot of the American Industrial Revolution. Henry David Thoreau dubbed it "the Manchester of America." The city was home to an unprecedented concentration of textile factories, which turned out high-quality cotton fabric. The busy mills were originally powered by water from a network of canals that ran through the city, driving waterwheels at forty factories that stretched for a mile along the Merrimack River. Those five-story brick buildings housed 320,000 spindles and almost ten thousand looms. At full production, the noise inside the mills was deafening.

And full production was the order of the day, at least at first. By 1846, Lowell was turning out just under a million yards of cloth a week; by 1850, its mills employed more than ten thousand workers, the majority of them women.[1] The first workers were local Yankee women from the countryside, but the mills soon needed more womanpower than the area could provide. That demand was met by immigrant labor. The first to arrive in Lowell were the Irish, beginning in the 1820s.

Since then, virtually every immigrant wave has left its imprint on the city. The Irish were followed by the French Canadians, the Greeks, and the Polish. Among the French Canadians were the parents of Lowell's most famous native son, Jack Kerouac. By 1910, Lowell's population also included Italians, Portuguese, Swedes, Armenians, Lithuanians, Russian Jews, and Syrians. From the end of World War II forward, even after the mills closed and the textile industry moved to the South, immigrants continued finding their way to Lowell.

About half of Lowell's current population consists of first-generation immigrants from Cambodia, Vietnam, Brazil, Portugal, Africa, and the Dominican Republic, as well as from Puerto Rico. Today, Lowell has the second largest Cambodian community in the United States. Lowell's history as a city of immigrants is reflected in the varied faces of its high school students. According to the *Lowell Sun,* 38 native languages are spoken by students at Lowell High School.[2] For almost half of all students, English is their second language. Twenty-five percent have limited proficiency in English.[3]

As school lets out, some teens quickly make their way toward a long line of buses queued up to transport them home. Even students on foot, however, do not tarry on the school grounds to say farewell to classmates; it is not permitted. Police officers in squad cars move assertively to disperse students, shouting through bullhorns and driving at close distance behind stragglers to encourage them to "move along" and "go home." In less than fifteen minutes, the campus is virtually deserted.

The heavy police presence at the high school and the insistent haste to clear the grounds is intended as a deterrent to gang activity, which in Lowell is no small problem. In a town of a little more than one hundred thousand people, there are eighteen thousand teens and young adults between the ages of thirteen and twenty-three. With twenty-five to thirty active gangs in the city, approximately 10 percent of those young people are gang-involved.[4] Most are the children of recently arrived immigrant groups.

Also present on the streets at dismissal time are several young adults in highly visible bright orange T-shirts or windbreakers. These individuals are members of the streetworker staff of Lowell's United Teen Equality Center (UTEC). As the students leave school, the streetworkers engage them in conversation, talking up UTEC's after-school programs and passing out leaflets inviting them to come play basketball, work out in the weight room, participate in dance workshops, use the computers, or just hang out. By giving young adults a better alternative to gang involvement,

UTEC and its streetworkers are in the forefront of local efforts to combat gang violence.

—∿— The UTEC Model

UTEC's motto is "Peace, Positivity, Empowerment." Serving nearly two thousand teens and young adults annually, UTEC "seeks to reduce risks that youth face day-to-day, increase opportunities for them to make positive changes in their lives and communities, and influence state and local policies that affect their ability to reach their potential."[5]

UTEC has four main programming areas: streetwork and peacemaking, education, youth development, and organizing and political action. Taken together, these four functions offer a healthy and productive way forward for at-risk young people, whose choices might otherwise be far more limited and far more dangerous. "Our four centers are the glue that holds everything together," says Jessica Wilson, UTEC director of development. "They are what make us different from other youth centers. Through streetworker outreach, even some young people who are the most disengaged can access all these different options here."

The name United Teen Equality Center was chosen by teenagers themselves, and equality is defined to mean not just equality among teens but also between teens and grown-ups. Every adult staff member works with a teen counterpart who has the same title and the same position. When it comes to a vote, everyone has equal power. Young people under the age of twenty-three also make up 50 percent of the board of directors. Richard Cavanaugh, a local attorney, is president of the UTEC board. "I've been involved with other nonprofits and other boards," he says, "and this is the first time I've ever been asked for a mood check at a meeting."

UTEC is teen run and teen led, a key factor that differentiates it from other service providers who "keep teens out of trouble" after school. Teens run all gatherings and special events, beginning with Circle Up. Summoned by the staccato rhythm of Survivor's "Eye of the Tiger" (the theme from *Rocky III*), every afternoon at 3:15, UTEC teens assemble around the game tables in the drop-in center for announcements. They drum up enthusiasm for their upcoming events, which run the gamut from a basketball game to culinary training to a poetry slam to a candidates' forum. (For the past five years, UTEC has hosted an evening for candidates running either for the school board or for the Lowell City Council. Teens moderate the well-attended event and select the questions for candidates to answer.)

By design, no one at UTEC is anonymous. "We have three staff members here at all times," says JuanCarlos Rivera, UTEC director of operations. "It's their responsibility to float around and to make sure teens are greeted personally as soon as they walk in. We're very intentional about that, and we're very intentional about making sure that folks remember other folks' names." To help them do so, UTEC staff members maintain and update a database of relevant information on all of their teens. "Young people really freak out when we remember their birthday, but for us it's a tool to give us the opportunity to have that interaction conversation." Born in Puerto Rico, Rivera has lived virtually all of his life in Lowell. Realizing at an early age that he wanted to work professionally with young people, he first became involved in community organizing through the Big Brothers Big Sisters program. After graduating from the University of Massachusetts at Lowell, he became one of UTEC's original staff members and was on hand when the doors opened for the first time.

—⁓— UTEC Beginnings

The beginnings of UTEC date from 1997. In the immediate aftermath of a gang incident between Latinos and Asians in which a young man was stabbed in the shoulder with a screwdriver, a group of teens organized themselves to take action. Pleading their case with the city, they emphasized that there was no safe place for them to gather in Lowell's downtown after school let out. (Downtown was already acknowledged by gang members as a "neutral zone.") It was not until 1999 that the teens marshaled enough support to enable UTEC to open its doors. Its first home was in the parish hall of St. Anne's Episcopal Church, next door to Lowell High School. The first day UTEC opened, it expected fifty teens; two hundred showed up.[6]

The center was a pioneering effort; it was Lowell's first collaborative venture that partnered a city agency, a neighborhood association, a local church, and a nonprofit service provider. Even so, UTEC's beginnings were extremely modest. The center opened with one part-time paid staff member, three volunteers, and an annual operating budget of $40,000. It took another year before UTEC was able to afford a paid leadership position. Gregg Croteau became executive director in February 2000 and remains its director today. With a B.A. from Wesleyan in East Asian studies, Croteau went on to complete his master's in social work at the University of Michigan, with a concentration on administration of nonprofit organizations. He has long had an interest in Southeast Asian culture; before heading up UTEC, he spent two years in Vietnam and is fluent in Vietnamese.

"UTEC's first step was to establish a safe haven for young people in the downtown area after school, but we knew that would be the first step of many to come," Croteau says. "We asked the teens in the center what they wanted. From their responses, we began to develop a plan that eventually became our four programming centers."

In 2003, UTEC applied to the Robert Wood Johnson Foundation Local Funding Partnerships program (at the time known as the Local Initiative Funding Partners program) for funding to support its streetworker gang intervention program. The fledgling agency had no difficulty documenting the need for its services. For a small city, the level of gang violence in Lowell was alarming. There had been twelve murders in 2002; there had also been sixteen gang-related shootings during an intensely violent five-month period.

Lowell has a relatively high crime rate compared with both the state of Massachusetts and the nation as a whole, and gang activity is largely responsible. Residents of Lowell are more than twice as likely as residents elsewhere to be victims of a violent personal crime such as rape, murder, assault, or robbery.[7] Active gang members make up almost 75 percent of gun homicide offenders and slightly less than half of all aggravated gun assault offenders.[8] According to the Lowell Police Department, young adults under the age of twenty commit 70 percent of all violent crimes in the city.[9]

"I remember UTEC's proposal quite clearly," recalls Pauline Seitz, program director of the Robert Wood Johnson Foundation Local Funding Partnerships program. "We always make it very clear to applicants that we do not extend the deadline; the only time we make an exception is when FEMA is in a community in response to a hurricane or other type of natural disaster. As the deadline arrived, I got a call from Gregg. He told us that UTEC's application would be unavoidably detained. 'FEMA is not in our neighborhood,' he began, 'but there was a shooting last night and we're surrounded by yellow police tape. We cannot leave to mail this to you, and FedEx cannot come in.'" Seitz approved the extension, but told Croteau to submit the application as soon as possible. When UTEC finally submitted its application, it was awarded $460,000 for a four-year period from July 2003 to June 2007. The Robert Wood Johnson Foundation grant funded the efforts of two outreach workers to reduce violence and improve teens' access to health care. The workers mediated gang conflicts, sponsored events and activities to promote peace, and established cooperative efforts with the police and other governmental partners to help abate gang violence.

—⁓— UTEC Relocates—Twice

At the time the Robert Wood Johnson grant was awarded, UTEC was still located within St. Anne's Episcopal Church. Early in the life of the grant, however, the church reclaimed the space for expanded religious programming. At that point, UTEC staff members began scrambling to find a stopgap location while urgently looking for a building to purchase as a permanent venue. Beginning in June 2004, the center's interim home was a cramped upstairs space in a storefront on Merrimack Street, close to the high school but smack in the heart of downtown.

This location soon brought UTEC into conflict with some downtown merchants who alleged that, as a magnet for at-risk and gang-involved youth, the center was driving up the crime rate and driving away customers.[10] In response, the center threw open its doors and invited skeptical business leaders inside to see what the teens were actually doing there. UTEC leaders held a large public meeting to answer questions and explain their philosophy and their programs. They also backed up their open door policy with hard statistical evidence from the Lowell Police Department, which showed that the crime rate had decreased after UTEC's establishment.[11]

"The approach we take to relationships is that no matter what happens, if someone makes derogatory comments about us, we are not going to react negatively," Gregg Croteau says. "After the church took back their space and our presence on Merrimack became an issue, we were challenged to respond. We decided very quickly that no matter what anyone said, we were going to remain positive, stay above it, and continue building relationships in the community."

The public nature of the conflict and the way in which the center dealt with it won UTEC many new supporters among residents and merchants alike. This powerful turnaround in public perception brought with it the solution to UTEC's relocation problem: an invitation from the much-diminished congregation of St. Paul's United Methodist Church, whose flock had dwindled down to its last seven parishioners. "The church contacted us because of the work we were doing and said, 'We would love you to be able to be in our home,'" recalls Rivera, an original staff member. "I love that expression, because it was their home, and we loved that they were sharing it." UTEC raised money to buy the church and completed the sale in February 2006.[12]

The spacious building accelerated the momentum initiated by the Robert Wood Johnson Foundation grant and facilitated a quantum leap forward for the organization. Simply put, the place took off. The Theodore Edson Parker Foundation, which is dedicated exclusively to supporting nonprofit organizations in the city of Lowell, was UTEC's nominating partner to the Robert Wood Johnson Foundation. "UTEC was this little scrappy agency; no one had any expectation that they could build what they did," says the Parker Foundation grant administrator, Phil Hall. "At the beginning, it was virtually impossible to imagine UTEC turning into the powerhouse it has become. Since the Robert Wood Johnson Foundation grant, it has been a chain of surprises from this group, all of them good."

Today, UTEC carries fifteen full-time staff members, nineteen part-time staff, and a budget of $2.2 million. It is supported by forty different funding institutions, including the City of Lowell, the Massachusetts Department of Public Health, the Massachusetts Executive Office of Public Safety and Security, the United States Department of Justice, the United States Department of Agriculture, the Amelia Peabody Foundation, the Roy A. Hunt Foundation, and the Bank of America.

"Without being hyperbolic, today it's well nigh inconceivable to be in this community and try to do anything constructive for kids without having UTEC at the table," says Judge Jay Blitzman, First Justice of the Middlesex County Juvenile Court. "UTEC has unusual credibility and currency with all sectors of the system . . . with the police, with the D.A., with the school system, with the courts, defense attorneys, prosecutors, and probation."

UTEC earned its reputation through a deliberate and consistent effort to build bridges both within Lowell and beyond it. The organization's staff, Gregg Croteau and JuanCarlos Rivera in particular, made connections with a wide range of city, state, and federal agencies, and with other service providers. "UTEC has done a remarkable job and has sustained a tremendous surge in growth," says Pauline Seitz.

—᪣— The Streetworker Program

The streetworker program remains at the core of UTEC's activities. At the beginning of the grant, the Robert Wood Johnson Foundation funding underwrote two paid streetworkers, who targeted seven of the most active gangs for intensive outreach. The initial concept was to use the city's basketball and volleyball courts to connect with gang-involved youth.

Almost immediately, however, it became clear that all other health and lifestyle issues had to remain secondary to waging peace; the urgent need was to stem the bloodshed between rival gangs. Tension was particularly high between Latino gangs, such as the Latin Kings, the Maniac Latin Disciples, and the Ñetas; and Asian groups, such as the Asian Boyz, the Tiny Rascal Gang, and the Blood Red Dragons. There was also violence among the Asian gangs themselves.

Many if not most of Lowell's Asian gangs are rooted in its sizeable Cambodian community, which numbers about thirty thousand, just under one-third of Lowell's entire population. Almost all first-generation Cambodians immigrated to the United States in the aftermath of that country's genocidal civil war. The brutal Pol Pot regime and the killing fields of the Khmer Rouge were responsible for the deaths of nearly two million Cambodians in the 1970s. During the 1980s, 114,000 survivors came to the United States as refugees.

Originally, refugees were dispersed and resettled in many different states. Eventually, however, they gravitated to a small number of Cambodian enclaves, including Lowell. At the time, work in the greater Boston area was relatively plentiful—this was the era of the Massachusetts Miracle, a period of robust economic growth centered on high-tech science and research firms along nearby Route 128. Lowell initially became a magnet for Cambodian expatriates because it had a concentration of markets where Cambodian food items were available and because there were a lot of under-the-table jobs in the area.

Although Cambodian refugees arrived with virtually no belongings, no one adequately comprehended the weight of the psychological baggage they were carrying. The degree to which they were traumatized in their homeland has become clear only in hindsight. In 2003, the National Institute of Mental Health and the National Institute on Alcohol Abuse and Alcoholism sponsored a study of Cambodian refugees. It found that 99 percent of respondents had nearly starved to death, 96 percent had been conscripted into forced labor, 90 percent had had a family member or friend murdered, and 54 percent had been tortured.[13] Because of these and other abuses, the overwhelming majority of Cambodians arrived in the United States with severe posttraumatic stress disorder (PTSD).

Sadly, this generation has never recovered. The study found that 62 percent met the diagnostic criteria for PTSD, even after more than two decades in the United States.[14] In addition to frequent flashbacks and nightmares that cause the sufferers to relive traumatic events over and over, common problems associated with chronic PTSD include emotional numbness, suicidal thoughts, explosive anger, passive-aggressive behavior, poor concentration, and persistent feelings of helplessness, shame, or guilt.

Because Cambodian teens and young adults have learned little if anything about the horrors of the Khmer Rouge from their elders, who were (and are) too shell-shocked to speak of their experiences, they have trouble coping with how PTSD manifests itself at home. Of necessity, many have had to assume adult responsibilities, even in early adolescence. They also have no meaningful way to grasp the dysfunctional effect PTSD has had on their family life, because the families of their friends are so much like their own.

Chronic PTSD has also exacerbated a cavernous cultural divide between the first and second generation of Cambodians. Although refugee Cambodians never assimilated into the community, their children were plunged headfirst into the American way of life. Their embrace of our popular culture stands in sharp contrast to the very traditional values of their parents, and has helped fuel a wrenching generational disconnect that remains painful and problematic to this day.

Cambodian parents keep their daughters close to home, or try to. "In our culture, if you're a girl and you're not at school, you're supposed to be at home cooking and cleaning. That's the way our parents were raised, and that's the only way our parents know how to raise children," says Sako Long, a veteran streetworker. Many Asian girls run away from home because they feel straitjacketed by the strictures their parents attempt to impose on them and believe they have no place to turn. "Most of the runaways we have in this community are Asian girls," Judge Blitzman says. "Their home life is oppressive." Once they get out on the street, they become vulnerable to overtures from gang members, who offer them food and shelter in exchange for sex and/or illicit activity. UTEC staff, together with other local social service providers, estimate that at any given time there are about three hundred homeless young people in Lowell. That's not counting the teens and young adults who may not be completely homeless, but who are sleeping on a different couch every night.

Adolescent Cambodian boys are given more physical freedom than their sisters, but are perhaps even more vulnerable to gang involvement. Their immersion in teen culture and their exposure to film, television, and music have fostered an appetite for glamour, bling, booze, and controlled substances. This desire for the material trappings of American prosperity greatly increases the allure of gang involvement. For a boy or young man already in conflict with his parents, part of the appeal of gangs is that they function like a substitute family. The gang will give him an identity, a sense of belonging, and a group of sympathetic individuals who will take his side and watch his back. "The glamorous life of a gang banger—the money, the jewelry, the fame: initially, the young person will see that and nothing more," Long says.

Only after the young recruit has tasted the pleasures of the gang lifestyle does he find out what it has cost him. "The gang leaders put it this way: 'We've given you all this. Now you have to give back,'" Rivera says. Typically, the first requests to "give back" will seem easy to do, like returning a favor. Often it may be something a teen will understand as a simple errand: "There's a package I need you to drop off. Don't worry about what's in it; just drop it off."

Intervening with adolescent boys and girls—ideally before they drop off that first package—is one of the fundamental missions of UTEC, and the streetworker program is at the heart of the center's approach to dealing with at-risk youth.

—⁓— Outreach and Intervention

Everything begins with outreach; streetworkers are highly proactive. They do not expect young people who need help will show up at the center. The streetworker presence at dismissal time at the high school is just one of many strategies. "We meet the teens where they're at," says the streetworker supervisor, Leslie Rivera.[15] "We don't wait for them to come to us; we go to them."

Streetworkers go out into the community every day, specifically to engage young people and build relationships with them. That can mean anything from going into the parks to play basketball, to being a presence at the movie theaters on a Friday evening, or to showing up at the emergency room after a teen has been wounded in a gang incident. Although UTEC does get referrals from the Department of Youth Services, from the schools, and from the courts, streetworkers also target neighborhoods where gang activity is prevalent. "We go house to house—literally door to door—to introduce ourselves to the community," Leslie Rivera says. "That way, the community feels comfortable with our being there; if there's a problem or a crisis, they will call on us to intervene."

Several times a month, these interventions become physical. When rival gang members are about to square off against one another, UTEC streetworkers literally place their bodies between them. "Any fight that there is in the city—it doesn't matter if we know you or not—as long as there is a fight and you look like a young person under the age of twenty-three, we're going to break it up," Leslie Rivera says. "I place myself sideways between the two individuals, so that they're facing my shoulder. I'm not face-to-face, so it's not confrontational. I'll say, 'We don't want you arrested. Let's go talk about this,' and even as we're talking, we'll be pushing the two individuals farther apart. We will separate the combatants first, and then find out what the problem is."

None of the streetworkers has ever been injured breaking up a fight. This is not only because of their training but also because of the credibility they have on the street. "We do a lot of intensive training to make sure that we're prepared," says JuanCarlos Rivera. "One misstep can change everything."

All streetworkers are from the community. Sako Long and several others are themselves former gang members. Others like Leslie Rivera have relatives who are still in gangs. "I'm somebody's aunt, somebody's cousin," she says. "If there's a problem with the Latin Kings or Latin Queens, it's easy for me to go talk to them. I don't have to work on building trust; they have known me for so long that trust is already there."

UTEC chose the color orange for streetworker uniforms because no gang uses it—and because it makes them stand out, both to the cops and to one another. "When we're dealing with a confrontation, I can look around and see at a glance how many streetworkers I have with me and where they are located," Leslie Rivera explains.

Spearheaded by Croteau and Lowell police superintendent Kenneth Lavallee, UTEC and the police have hammered out an understanding and a rapport. "We now have a very solid partnership with UTEC," says Lavallee. "Members of UTEC staff and representatives of the police department, including members of our gang unit, meet on a regular basis. We have developed a great working relationship with UTEC, and it has improved over the years."

"It's important that the officers understand the work that streetworkers do, and that we respect the work that the police do," says JuanCarlos Rivera. "We don't always agree, but the fact that we have constant communication is extremely important."

Not surprisingly, the perspective of the Lowell Police Department stems from its mission to protect public safety, not just of young adults but of all citizens. Sworn officers, for example, cannot be expected to look away from a physical gang confrontation; they will step in and make arrests. The opportunity streetworkers have is to break it up before the cops arrive.

The UTEC perspective is rooted in its commitment to problem solving and life enhancement for each individual teen and young adult. UTEC puts this belief into practice within its own staff. Many started as clients of the agency, and several key staff members have extensive prior gang involvement. Sako Long had joined a Lowell street gang at the age of thirteen; at eighteen, he was sent up to the Billerica House of Correction on a series of gun charges. His time in jail listening to the screams of other prisoners being raped or beaten pushed him to leave the gang lifestyle behind. Today Long is UTEC's director of athletics. "Many cops think once you're a gang member, you're always a gang member," says Superintendent Lavallee. "That's not true. Sako gave me a very powerful lesson about turning his life around. It was very enlightening to me, and it's a message a lot of people should hear."[16]

—ᴍ— Relationship Building and Problem Solving

Paradoxically, intervention to stop a fight is one of UTEC's best opportunities to make a difference in a young person's life. Streetworkers who have broken up a fight continue their relationship with those involved. When they place their bodies between rival gang members, streetworkers are in effect taking on new clients—and taking on a serious commitment to help them.

"They become part of our caseload," Leslie Rivera says. "We do the follow-up, make phone calls, get to know who their support network is. We learn who the people are in their lives that they trust, and build relationships with them as well. We become more like family." At any given time, each streetworker has a caseload of approximately thirty young adults.

Even after UTEC gets gang-involved teens into the center, however, it can still be difficult to get them to open up about challenges they may be having. One key UTEC staff member in this effort is Elena Ansara, a social worker who is employed by the Mental Health Association for Greater Lowell. Ansara spends afternoons and evenings at UTEC when the center is open. Her job begins by hanging out—by having conversations with teens without letting them know she's a social worker. Those ostensibly casual conversations often lead to one-on-one counseling sessions. "Elena is invaluable," JuanCarlos Rivera says. "In addition to counseling young people, she is present in team meetings, coaching the rest of our staff on how best to approach various sensitive issues. Our streetworkers will take Elena with them on home visits whenever someone's been kicked out of the house or there's been a death or a suicide attempt."

"Crisis is opportunity," says Croteau. "UTEC sees every crisis as an opportunity for intervention, a chance to get involved with a young person, not a chance to step away. We can engage them in positive activities based on their interests or help solve problems that to teens may seem insurmountable." Problem solving is how streetworkers tap into the other three programming areas UTEC offers: education, youth development, and organizing and political action.

"We call them the hooks," says JuanCarlos Rivera, "because they enable us to maintain and expand our relationships with gang-involved and at-risk young people." And UTEC has developed a lot of hooks, many more than when the Robert Wood Johnson Foundation grant program first started.

Among them is UTEC's Open School program. Many gang members have dropped out of school or are on the verge of doing so. "In Massachusetts, the data show that 50 percent of all students who have not graduated from high school will be arrested by the time they are thirty years old," Judge Blitzman says. "That's a heartbreaking statistic."

Lowell High School has a four-year graduation rate of 69.5 percent, which places it in the bottom 10 percent of all high schools in the state of Massachusetts. UTEC offers two separate programs for those whose high school education is incomplete. One is a standard GED program. The other is an Alternative Diploma Program (ADP), in partnership with Lowell High School. Most students in this program have had to drop out or leave school for a couple of months, whether because of situations at home or at work, or for personal reasons, such as illness, incarceration, or pregnancy. When they are able to resume their education, the public school system does not have any mechanism that would allow the students to pick up where they left off. If they leave partway through the school year, they must start over the following September and repeat the grade they were in. With the UTEC program, those months are not wasted. Students who complete their high school education through ADP earn a Lowell High School diploma and are entitled to go to the prom and "walk" with their fellow graduating classmates.

Lola Akintobi is UTEC's Open School coordinator, and works with both the GED and the ADP programs. In addition to helping young people earn their high school diplomas, she also works to broaden their horizons by showing that the diploma should not be the end of their education. "In our UTEC class called Life Choices and Possibilities, we go through all the skills the students will need after graduation—skills that don't necessarily get taught in a high school setting," she says. "We teach students how to prepare a résumé, how to fill out a job application, how to complete a college application, how to find a college or trade school, and how to determine whether it fits your needs. Then we work with each student one on one to set up a plan specifically for them."

UTEC's youth development programming is wide-ranging and includes art, cultural, and sports programs, but not all programming in this division is recreational. Teens can also learn useful skills such as basic computer literacy and Web design. Key to many older teens is job training. UTEC's popular Fresh Roots program provides jobs and job training to help teens enter the workforce in the food and beverage industry. Derek Mitchell is UTEC's Fresh Roots coordinator. He explains that "a lot of young people, if you have tattoos on your arm, if you're nineteen years old and you've never had a 'check job,' as the teens call them—meaning a job that's not under the table—it's really hard to break into the job market, especially with times as they are. We want young people to develop a real skill; we want to provide that initial foot in the door. More than that, we want to provide a leg up to give a young person an opportunity to manage a program and a business, which is really empowering."

"There's a girl here in the Fresh Roots program who's been to five different high schools," says UTEC board president Richard Cavanaugh, "and in the course of her high school years, she's never graduated. She found a home here, and she's been baking. I am enthusiastic about this place because they're taking a life that so easily could go one way, and they are changing it around."[17]

UTEC's youth organizing programs are intended to increase young people's awareness of their own political power and their ability to make a difference in bringing about lasting social change. Issues can be local, such as getting Lowell's buses to run later in the evening, or broader, such as advocating for more funding for teen pregnancy prevention programs. UTEC's track record in this regard is mixed. Despite requests by UTEC teens to extend the bus schedule to 8:00 P.M. nightly, Lowell Regional Transit

Authority buses still end their runs at 7:00 P.M. However, the teen advocates have had far more success at the state level with regard to preserving funding for teen pregnancy prevention. Although the state legislature has attempted to cut the allocation in half in each of the past three years, UTEC's call and letter writing campaign is credited with helping get the program funded.

One program component is called Teens Leading the Way. It is a statewide coalition of young people who learn the political process and learn to use public policy to address teen health issues. Among UTEC's young people active in Teens Leading the Way is Eddie Mercado, who had been an active member of the Chicago-based Maniac Latin Disciples since the age of fourteen. Now twenty, Mercado is no stranger to gang violence. In 2004, two close cousins were killed in front of their home in a drive-by shooting. Their murders left him with a sense of despair and rage that propelled him into gang life. "I used to be the first one to start something," he says. "People were scared of me here in Lowell because of what I used to do."

Mercado has been stabbed three times, and one of those stabbings nearly killed him; it took the paramedics five minutes to revive him. Mercado woke up in a hospital bed and needed months of rehabilitation to relearn how to walk and speak correctly. By the time friends brought him to UTEC, he had already dropped out of high school. "Because of what had happened to my cousins, I was really paranoid," he says. "It took me awhile to develop a relationship with the streetworkers and the UTEC staff, but they kept showing me they cared. They got me back on my feet; they got me a job. Then they encouraged me to get involved in policy making and organizing. I went through teen leadership training, and I started working with Gregg. Now I'm almost done with my alternative diploma. From there, I'm jumping into college, probably in political science or criminal justice. I'm also involved in the Statewide Youth Council. Governor Deval Patrick knows me very well."

For his contributions, Mercado received a Rising Star Volunteer Award from the Greater Lowell Community Foundation. However, he is technically still a member of the Maniac Latin Disciples—not his choice. "The streetworkers tried getting me out, but I'm still in by blood," he explains. "I was sworn for life. I know if I go to Chicago, I'm going to get jumped or killed. To them, I'm a disgrace."[18]

—᠆ᡵᡳ— Peacemaking

Using the trust they have built up with gang-involved young people, UTEC streetworkers approach them about participating in the peacemaking process.[19] This process begins within a gang before it ever happens between gangs. Streetworkers invite as many as twenty members of the same set to join them on a peace trip. "But we don't call it a peace trip. It's much more casual than that," Leslie Rivera says. "We say, 'We're going out—do you guys want to come along?'"

"We try to do something fun that gets them out of their comfort zone and away from their surroundings," Anthony Ellis, a UTEC streetworker, says.

"We take them bowling, which they've never done, or go-carting, or fishing," says Sako Long. "Fishing is one of the things I love to do with young people—it's a chance to kick back, and it's a great time for us to communicate and relax. It's a peaceful day, with a lot of conversation.

"While we're there, we'll start to talk about the streets with them," Long continues. "More often than not, they'll tell us they've been having problems with another gang. I tell them my story, that I lived their lifestyle before and that I've been out of it for a long time. Then I ask, 'How would you feel if you had just one less enemy?' This question really hits home, because right now they're watching their back every minute. They can't walk down the street without worrying about getting followed.

By getting them to think about having fewer enemies, this is how we plant the seed of peace."

After one or more peace trips, the step that follows is a peace circle. Before then, however, the streetworkers meet to strategize. "We discuss who will participate," says JuanCarlos Rivera. "We choose ten; in general, they will be the ones with some leadership role who seemed most likely to be receptive to what we're trying to do."

"The peace circle is a Native American way of communicating," Long says. "Within the circle, we talk about respect and what it means to each individual. The young men share their life stories and talk about the serious issues that are affecting them. Everyone feels a little awkward at first, but it becomes very powerful as soon as these young people hear their friends talking about the problems in their lives."

"When you're at the superficial level where you're drinking and talking about women and the Red Sox and this and that, it's not really deep conversation," Rivera says. "Often this is the first time they've opened up to their friends. We've had gang members who have busted out crying, who have shared information that is extremely personal to them. That's the breakthrough for us."

Up to this point, the peacemaking process has taken place on parallel tracks with two separate gang sets. The streetworkers hold separate peace trips and peace circles within two gangs before ever trying to bring the rivals together. Not every peace circle leads to a peace summit. The young gang members have to have a certain degree of openness before streetworkers will suggest it. When they take place, however, they bring a lasting benefit to the community as a whole and to the young men themselves.

Streetworkers again confer and strategize about who should be invited. "We are looking for a circle of no more than ten, five from each set," says JuanCarlos Rivera, "and we are looking for the decision makers. We know them as shot callers." The shot callers are often reluctant. "'What have you got to lose?' I ask," says Long. "'Give it a chance—talk to this other gang. If it doesn't work out, you're in no worse shape than you are now. And if it does work out, you'll have one less enemy to deal with.'"

To maximize the appeal of the summit, streetworkers offer the chance for a true outdoor adventure, an entire weekend away from Lowell, often something with an adrenalin rush. "We've done kayaking, whitewater rafting, things that urban teens have never tried," Long says. "When we give them that opportunity, they're really excited about the prospect.... "

"At least until our van pulls up with five members of a rival set inside," Gregg Croteau adds. "On the trip out of town, there's often absolute silence—for five hours."

Streetworkers sit between the rival sets. "Even though they know they're going on this weekend to talk about peace, they all have second thoughts at the beginning," Long says. "Once we get to our destination, we get them involved in some structured activities. We'll give them icebreakers and team builders that get them talking together, laughing together, and working together. We have them do food exercises, so they cook with each other. It's our job to get them to feel a little bit better about this whole situation."

By the time the streetworkers bring the rivals around the campfire for a joint peace circle, the young men are more at ease, more open to sharing their stories. In one key part of the process, streetworkers ask each person around the circle to list the five things that matter most to him, and then to name the one thing that's most important of all. "And 99 percent of the time it's about family," Long says. "So we talk about what family means to each of them." As the rivals go around the circle, they are amazed, because all of them are going through pretty much the same thing, and the young men come to realize they are not so different from one another after all. "Once they've shared these kinds of stories, it's very hard for them to still think of the others around the campfire as the enemy," Long says.

That is essential to the adventure component of the weekend—the activity they had all been looking forward to.

Streetworkers intentionally set up the adventure so that it requires cooperation and teamwork between the two gang sets. They have paired up rival shot callers in a two-man kayak. If they don't work together, they're upside down in the rapids—together—and that's precisely the point.

Sam Man was a gang member who went through the peacemaking process. With the help and encouragement of streetworkers, he learned to complete a résumé and got a job. He had already been shot and seriously wounded. "I could have been locked up," he says. "Every time I was in court, they were there with me. I've got friends who are doing life right now. I've got friends that died. I could have died. They did me a big favor."

After several fishing trips with Sako Long, Man agreed to participate in a whitewater rafting summit. "It was us and some Latin guys," Man says. "I don't like him because he's Latino. He doesn't like me because I'm Asian. I thought we would just be able to do the trip and stay in our own individual groups, but they set us up. They put our group and their group together in one raft. If we didn't work as a team, everybody was going to drown."

The peace summit closes with a fire ceremony, during which each participant leaves something behind and takes something away. Each young man writes something on a piece of paper that symbolizes what he is abandoning, and then throws the paper into the fire. What each of them take away is a commitment to peace with the others who have been on the weekend adventure. "That commitment is quite specific," Long says. "We are very straightforward to say that the treaty applies only to those present, not to their entire gang. Nevertheless, for each of them, that's five fewer enemies that they have."

The peacemaking process has evolved and strengthened during the past several years. Ongoing streetworker outreach, together with enforcement efforts by the Lowell Police Department, appears to be generating measurable results. "Over the past several years, there has been a reduction in gang violence in

Lowell, particularly in homicide," says Superintendent Lavallee. "In 2006, there were fourteen murders in Lowell. We've seen a steady reduction since then. In the three years that followed, we've had fewer homicides combined than in that one single year. I attribute that reduction to the work we've done together to prevent gang violence."

—⟅⟆— The Future of UTEC

Today UTEC is not only sustainable but poised for additional growth. "The vision I have for the future is the vision I've witnessed," says the board president, Richard Cavanaugh. "My hope is that now that UTEC has grown to the size it is, we can start to do a better job with some of the more mundane organizational issues, while making sure that none of the spirit is lost. I'm here to try to make the trains run on time, and not in any way discourage the great ideas that keep bubbling up from our teens. I also see my role as helping to spread the story about UTEC to get other people involved."

The staff is well aware of problems that can ensue when an organization grows too fast. "We've seen too many agencies fall into a trap," Croteau says. "They get a big splash and then cannot sustain it. We're still early in our development. UTEC just celebrated its tenth anniversary, but it feels as though we're really more like a five- or six-year-old agency, because we started so small. We intend to be around for a long time, and we want to be really intentional about the idea of expanding in any way."

Future plans include expansion of the streetworker program, including establishment of a Streetworker Training Institute that would teach other agencies how to implement its peacemaking model and that has the potential to become a revenue generator for UTEC. Renovations to the headquarters building have already been designed and are in the approval process. New facilities will include a dance studio, sound recording and video production facilities, and more classroom space, plus an additional 7,500 square feet of new construction that will house a café and a catering operation to expand the very successful Fresh Roots program. When completed, UTEC's 20,000-square-foot headquarters will also be a LEED (Leadership in Energy and Environmental Design)–certified building. In April 2010, UTEC was awarded $1.9 million in federal stimulus money for the new construction. Groundbreaking for the new building was expected to take place by the end of 2010.

"We talk about the success of UTEC in terms of individual stories, but we need to be able to show it statistically," Croteau says. "We have hired an evaluation director, because we want to focus on being an outcomes-based agency." And the Johns Hopkins Bloomberg School of Public Health is evaluating the streetworker program and is developing a model showing how the streetworker program affects youth violence.

The evaluation tools "will not only help us document our progress with potential funders but will also help us in-house as well," Croteau says. "We always want to continue to improve, to learn from what works and how we can tweak it to make it work better. Whatever best practices are out there, we can adapt to our situation, and whatever best practices we have developed can be written up and shared with a wider audience."

What is far more difficult to quantify and to impart to others, however, is the remarkable sense of dedication exhibited by UTEC staff. "What they do is very tough," Sandy Lopacki, former deputy director of the Local Initiative Funding Partners program, says, "but there has been virtually no turnover. They are very deep in terms of staff who are committed to the mission of UTEC. The staff stays there and they figure out ways to reward them beyond just a salary increase."

"I attended a celebration dinner, and on the table at every seat was the picture of a teen with a short story about how his or her life had been changed by UTEC," Lopacki continues.

Lopacki points to Johnny Chheng as one of the agency's biggest success stories. "I started at UTEC when they were first in St. Anne's," Chheng says. "Streetworkers found me in the park, helped me get a copy of my birth certificate, helped me get my social security number, and then a job. Even so, when I was sixteen, I got involved with gang issues, deeply active. I was living a life I didn't want to lead, but I knew I couldn't leave. I was in too deep. I committed a serious crime—I nearly killed somebody—and I got locked up for five years." "All the time I was inside, the streetworkers visited me, called me on the phone," he continues. "Gregg sent me books to read. When I got out, Sako was there. 'We've got a reentry plan for you,' he told me. 'We've got stuff for you to do.'"

Today Johnny Chheng is a volunteer on UTEC's staff through the AmeriCorps program; he is an outreach specialist in training to become a streetworker. Part of his job is to help teens who have been given community service hours by the courts get into one of UTEC's community service programs. "Now I feel like I can put my experience to work helping other teens. Every time I go to sleep, I feel good about myself. It's time for me to give back in a positive way, because they never gave up on me."

Notes

1. National Park Service. *Lowell: The Story of an Industrial City.* Washington, D.C.: Government Printing Office, 2001, p. 39.
2. Scott, C. "Bienvenidos and Welcome." *Lowell Sun,* May 6, 2007.
3. Massachusetts Department of Education for Elementary and Secondary Education, School District Profiles. "Lowell High (01600505)." 2010. http://profiles.doe.mass.edu/profiles/student.aspx?orgcode=01600505& orgtypecode=6&leftNavId=300&.
4. UTEC staff interview with Lowell Police Department superintendant Kenneth Lavallee, March 12, 2008.
5. United Teen Equality Center. *Prospectus.* Lowell, Mass.: United Teen Equality Center, 2008, p. 5.
6. Savard, R. "Saving Teens for 10 Years." *Lowell Sun,* November 7, 2009. http://utec-lowell.org/press/pdf/11_07_09.jpg.

7. CLRsearch.com. "Demographics for Lowell, MA." 2010. http://www
   .clrsearch.com/RSS/Demographics/MA/Lowell/.

8. McDevitt, J., Braga, A. A., and Cronin, with S., McGarrell, E. F., and
   Bynum, T. "Project Safe Neighborhoods: Strategic Interventions, Lowell,
   District of Massachusetts, Case Study 6," February 2007, pp. 9–10.
   http://www.ojp.usdoj.gov/BJA/pdf/Lowell_MA.pdf.

9. UTEC staff interview with Lowell Police Department superintendant
   Kenneth Lavallee, March 12, 2008.

10. Scott, C. "Loitering Teens Are Hurting Us." *Lowell Sun.* December 13,
    2004. http://www.utec-lowell.org/press/pdf/img006.jpg.

11. Scott, C. "Stats Show Teens Not Causing Rise in Crime Downtown."
    Lowell Sun, December 19, 2004, http://www.utec-lowell.org/press/pdf/
    img007.jpg.

12. St. Paul's is an 1839 Greek Revival structure. As part of the conversion
    process, UTEC auctioned the massive pipe organ on eBay, but not before
    hosting one farewell organ concert in the sanctuary. The concert drew
    many longtime residents, who told stories of their own weddings and
    baptisms in the church to the UTEC teens, in effect passing the torch to
    the next generation.

13. National Institute of Mental Health. "PTSD, Depression Epidemic
    Among Cambodian Immigrants." August 2005. http://www.nimh.nih
    .gov/science-news/2005/ptsd-depression-epidemic-among-cambodian-
    immigrants.shtml.

14. Marshall, G., and others. "Mental Health of Cambodian Refugees
    Two Decades After Resettlement in the United States." *Journal of the
    American Medical Association,* 2005, *294.* http://jama.ama-assn.org/cgi/
    content/full/294/5/571.

15. Leslie Rivera and JuanCarlos Rivera are not related.

16. Sako is one of the subjects of a new documentary film about gang violence.
    Titled *On Track,* it describes Sako's experiences as well as those of two
    other former gang members. Produced by the Middlesex County District
    Attorney's Office with financing from the U.S. Department of Justice, the
    film will be distributed to schools across Massachusetts.

17. Fresh Roots also takes young people out to work on an organic farm to
    reinforce their connection to the process of growing and harvesting food.
    For further information, visit http://www.worldvisionreport.org/Blogs/
    Teen-Farmers and http://www.worldvisionreport.org/special_report/
    Fresh-Roots-Organic-Farm.

18. Mercado has made a video telling his story, available at http://
    www.youtube.com/watch?v=74Nqim6-0PU.

19. A brief music video outlines the services streetworkers provide and
    how services lead into the peace process. Go to http://www.youtube
    .com/watch?v=kVLImxu-EH8.

CHAPTER 6

Dental Health Aides and Therapists in Alaska

Sara Solovitch

Editors' Introduction

How to deliver health care services to people living in remote areas has long been a challenge to health policy planners. One way, of course, is to offer incentives so that highly trained professionals will locate in remote places. Another is to train health professionals from rural areas in the expectation that they will return home or to another rural location after completing their training. A third way is to train less highly qualified health professionals who are more likely to settle and work in a remote area. This is the approach that the Robert Wood Johnson Foundation adopted in the 1970s to develop the professions of nurse practitioners and physicians' assistants who would then be expected to practice in underserved, especially rural, areas. A fourth approach is to give a limited amount of training to members of the community, who then can provide basic services to their neighbors. This model is used widely in underdeveloped countries, most famously with China's barefoot doctors, and more sparingly in the United States.

Alaska is a huge state with inhospitable terrain. Many of its villages are accessible only by planes flown by bush pilots (and even then, only when the villages are not snowed in). Moreover, the health of its inhabitants, particularly of Alaska Natives, ranks among the very lowest in the nation. Tooth decay, which is a very serious problem among poor people generally, is an especially critical problem in Alaska, and it is exacerbated by a lack of dentists who live in or visit remote communities.

To remedy the problem, the Rasmuson Foundation, and later the W.K. Kellogg Foundation, instituted a program to train a new class of health personnel, dental therapists. Students received two years of training in New Zealand, which had pioneered the concept of dental therapists, and then returned to their communities to provide basic dental services. This aroused the ire of the Alaska Dental Society and the American Dental Association, which sued to put a stop to what they considered to be inadequately trained individuals practicing dentistry. The aftereffects of the conflict between organized dentistry and those promoting the idea of midlevel personnel offering basic dental services reverberates today.

In this chapter, award-winning journalist Sara Solovitch chronicles the history of dental therapists and dental aides in Alaska. The chapter is unlike most others in the *Anthology* series in that the Robert Wood Johnson Foundation played only a small role in the story. In 2004, the Foundation, through its Local Initiative Funding Partners program, awarded the Alaska Native Tribal Health Consortium a grant to train a new category of dental practitioners called *dental health aides*. Dental health aides would receive two weeks of training and be able to offer very basic services, such as patient education and fluoride rinses. The Foundation later made a small grant to enable officials of the American Dental Association to fly to rural Alaska to see the dental health aides and dental health therapists in action.

Even though the Robert Wood Johnson Foundation's role was tangential, the story is still an important one. As recently as the health reform debate of 2009 and 2010, Congress was wrestling with the question of whether people without dentistry degrees should be permitted to offer oral health services in communities not served by dentists.

Jackson is only eight years old, but he works like a little man, packing water and hauling wood each day at home in Kiana, a village of four hundred people just north of the Arctic Circle. When his family go out on their boat—they are Inupiat Eskimos, whose life on the Alaskan tundra revolves around hunting, fishing, and berry picking—Jackson is always first to reach for the anchor. Come evening, he is the one who prepares the kindling for his great-grandmother's morning fire—a good boy whose worth is already evident, as his grandmother notes, by the calluses on his hands.

But on a recent mild September morning, those small, calloused hands are cradling a badly bulged-out cheek, swollen to twice its size from a tooth blackened with decay. Jackson sits in the single dentist's chair at Kiana's health clinic, staring straight ahead at the cinderblock walls, plainly willing himself not to cry.

Toothache is no stranger to Jackson; it has been an unwelcome and intermittent presence as long as he can remember. At the age of two, he was airlifted 550 miles to a hospital in Anchorage, where his four front baby teeth were extracted under general anesthesia. Just three months ago in July, he sat in this very chair as three of his permanent molars—black and rotted—were removed. And now this.

"It started hurting the other night," says his grandmother, Janet, who had been outside her house cutting caribou when Jackson's teacher called to report that he was in too much pain to stay in school. "He was chewing on some dried meat when it started hurting."

"Must have been some good *paniqtaq*, eh?" commiserates Kimberly Baldwin, the dental therapist who just a few months ago took out Jackson's molars. Jackson gives a slight uplift of the eyebrows—a quintessential Inupiaq way of saying yes—and Baldwin tries looking in his mouth, past his few remaining baby teeth, all capped with stainless steel. No luck. The infection is too far gone. The boy can't open wide enough to let her see inside. He'll need an antibiotic to reduce the inflammation before anyone can poke around and pull another tooth.

Baldwin herself isn't authorized to prescribe antibiotics; she is part of a small cadre of Alaskan dental therapists who have been trained to drill and fill cavities, extract teeth, perform X-rays, apply fluoride varnishes and sealants, and give instruction to prevent tooth decay. She works under the supervision of a dentist who regularly reviews her patient charts and, in cases like Jackson's, orders the necessary prescriptions. That dentist is usually based at the Maniilaq Health Center, the hub hospital in Kotzebue that is about sixty miles away, and is available via telemedicine hookup.

Baldwin herself grew up a few miles downriver from Kiana in a village called Noorvik and was raised on a traditional diet and a subsistence way of life. A petite thirty-one year old who could easily pass for twenty-one, she sprinkles her conversation with Inupiat words the way a New Yorker uses Yiddish. She and her husband, who works at the local zinc mine, are determined to pass on the old ways to their two young daughters.

Kiana is home, and Baldwin is quick to point out its natural beauty. It's a rough and beautiful spot on the Kobuck River, a place that catches the winds whipping off the Chukchi Sea just ten miles distant. The houses are built on pilings to separate them from the permafrost, permanently frozen ground. By September, the caribou migration has begun and all through town the animals' butchered legs hang drying from house beams. The land, seen from the air, is the color of toasted wheat; at ground level, the hues are subtle and rich. The tundra is bursting with blackberries, cranberries, and a low-growing shrub called tundra tea, which is reputed to be filled with healthful properties. Baldwin knows all the best picking spots.

Less than a block from the clinic, several small boys crouch in silence as a seventy-four-year-old woman, dressed in an *aitikluk,* the traditional Inupiat woman's smock, bends over a freshly shot wolf. "There's a lot of fat," the woman remarks, flaying open the wolf's belly under Baldwin's critical eye. The animal, killed by the woman's grandson at the village dump, is lying flat on its back on a pallet, its legs distended to the endless sky, its enormous white teeth locked in a perfect bite. "He's been eating a lot of caribou."

Members of the high school cross country team run past in pairs, indifferent to the wolf skinning. A small electric coil sends up a whiff of smoke; it's intended to keep flies off the carcass, but they're congregating in ever-greater numbers. The little boys still haven't moved from their perch.

When, after about twenty minutes, the grandmother, or *ana,* as Baldwin calls her, complains that her back is aching, Baldwin offers to finish the job. Immediately, it's apparent that here is someone who knows how to skin a wolf. Under her knife, the thick fur slides off the femur; the bushy tail pulls away from its muscle. And all the while the wolf's blood is silently dripping off the pallet, drenching her pants legs. At last, the skinning is complete, and Baldwin stands up and looks at her watch. It's time to clean up, go back to the clinic, and see her next patient.

—∿— Oral Health in Alaska

Dental therapists like Kim Baldwin are a relatively new addition to Alaskan health care. Midlevel providers, they operate under the auspices of the Community Health Aide Program (CHAP), which was authorized by Congress in 1968 to train villagers to provide medical care in remote Alaska. The impetus was the 1950s tuberculosis epidemic, when TB was at its peak (morbidity rates from TB in the 1950s were the highest ever reported in the medical literature),[1] and the mortality rate of Native children was more than one hundred times that of children in the Lower 48.[2] Today there are approximately 550 health aides working in more than 170 villages across the state, acting essentially like the legendary barefoot doctors of China—mending broken legs, delivering vaccinations, assisting in childbirth, and responding to all matter of trauma, from suicide to fire to snowmobile accidents.

They form the backbone of rural Alaska Native health care and provide more than 350,000 patient visits each year.

Today's oral health crisis in Alaska has sparked numerous comparisons with the TB epidemic of the 1950s, but it is hardly unique to Alaska. A "silent epidemic of oral diseases" is a national problem, first brought to light in a 2000 landmark report by the United States Surgeon General titled *Oral Health in America.*[3] Among the findings: Tooth decay is the most common chronic childhood disease, interfering with daily activities for an estimated four million to five million children and adolescents each year.[4]

Still, the problem is far grimmer in Alaska than anywhere else in the United States, except perhaps on Indian reservations. In Alaska, the real measure for disease is untreated lesions, cavities that go untreated for months or longer for lack of oral care. According to a 1999 survey by the Indian Health Service, untreated lesions exist in 68 percent of American Indian and Alaska Native adolescents, compared to 24 percent of other children in the United States.[5]

Anecdotally, the number today is believed to be even greater. One-third of Alaska Native children report missing some days of school each year because of dental pain. Half of all Native kids under three undergo general anesthesia for extraction of their baby teeth, and it is commonplace to see schoolchildren with mouths full of metal.

In the Kiana health clinic, Baldwin keeps a plastic bag filled with the hundreds of teeth she has extracted—Jackson's among them. And one doesn't have to be a dentist to see at a glance that all of the teeth are seriously diseased; one after the other is marked with large black and brown grooves and holes. As Baldwin puts it, "The abnormal is normal here. Things we saw in the textbook that we were told were rare, that we'd never see, we see all the time."

This wasn't always the case. Physical anthropologists of the last century rhapsodized over the perfect, healthy teeth they discovered in that remote part of the world. In a 1939 classic text, *Nutrition and Physical Degeneration*, dentist Weston A. Price, who has been called the "Charles Darwin of Nutrition," declared oral health in Alaska to be among the best in the world. Recent archaeological digs confirm that dental caries simply didn't exist among the Inupiats and Yupiks of a thousand years ago. If anything, those coastal people had teeth worn down to the gum line—a result of a lifetime of chewing tough, dried meat. But the wear and tear also came from using their teeth as a tool. Inupiat women chewed the skin of bearded seals to soften hides for boots and crimp the toes and heels, and men used their teeth to bend wood to form the interior ribs of kayaks.

Those ways mostly stopped after World War II, as supply lines opened and a Western diet gradually supplanted the traditional Native foods. By the 1950s, a ship called the *North Star* sailed yearly up the Alaskan coast, carrying supplies and boxes of candy, along with a doctor and a dentist on board.

"Elders would row the kids out to the boat and there would be one line on deck to get inoculations and another line for the dentist to take out your teeth," recounts Mark Kelso, a public health dentist with the Norton Sound Health Corporation who still speaks with a Texan twang, although he has been practicing twenty-three years in Nome. "That established a regional concept of dentistry in some families that still exists today, that was thoroughly ingrained when I came here.... You don't see a dentist till you're in pain."

Today a high-sugar diet has become so entrenched that many public health nurses, doctors, dentists, and therapists recall being bumped off a bush plane on its way to a remote village to make room for a shipment of soda pop, candy, and Pop-Tarts. Soda pop is a village staple. A survey by dentists of the Norton Sound Health Corporation in the mid-1980s determined average soda consumption in that northern coastal region to be six cans per person per day.[6] "And I can tell you from observation that that's still the case," Kelso says.

Even villagers who know better—dental therapists in training, for example—say they find it hard to withstand the sugar onslaught. Fredella Sharp, a dental therapist in training, says she breastfed her older daughter for a year in Fairbanks before moving back to the village, where the child's grandparents spoiled her with unlimited soda. "All her teeth are silver," Sharp says shyly. "We went to Dillingham and she was tied down in the dentist's office and had her teeth pulled. I was really mad at their dad. I told him the next time one of our kids had to go through this he was going to go with them. 'Cause I wasn't going to do it again."

The effects of poor diet are exacerbated by a bacterium, *Streptococcus mutans,* which has been identified in Alaska Natives at levels many times that of the general population. *S. mutans* lives in the mouth, thrives on sugar, and gives off an acid that wears away tooth enamel and causes caries. Widely recognized as a primary cause of tooth decay, it is transmitted directly by mother or primary caregiver—often by blowing on the child's food. In Alaskan tribal culture, mothers and grandmothers customarily chew food before passing it directly into the child's mouth—a surefire way of spreading this mouth-borne bacterium.

Making matters worse is the lack of access to care. In 1998, a white paper by Tom Bornstein, dental director of the SouthEast Alaska Regional Health Consortium in Juneau, revealed that only twenty or so dentists served the state's more than two hundred far-flung villages inhabited by a total of 85,000 people. That's a ratio of one dentist to every 4,250 people. Bornstein presented his paper the following year at a meeting of the dental directors of the recently formed Alaska Native Tribal Health Consortium (ANTHC). His paper is generally credited as the original impulse behind the dental therapy program.

In the past decade, the Denali Commission, an independent federal agency charged with building medical and municipal infrastructure across Alaska, has partnered with entities throughout the state to build nearly one hundred state-of-the-art health clinics, including the one in Kiana. Many of the state's remaining one hundred or so villages are not large enough to sustain their own independent clinic. So, for example, when dentists from the Southcentral Foundation, a Native-owned health care organization based in Anchorage, make their twice-yearly pilgrimage by bush plane to each of the twenty-four villages in their jurisdiction, they carry thousands of pounds of gear: drills, X-ray machine and processor, chairs, lights, and compressor. They set up shop wherever they can water and find the space, sometimes in the school gym, sometimes in a storage space. Occasionally they manage to find a bed for the night, but just as often they sleep on a table or on the floor.

Volunteer dentists have also been flying up to Alaska for years—interspersing patient visits with time out for hunting and fishing.

Tribal leaders say that's all very nice, but hardly a long-term solution for an oral care crisis of Alaskan proportions. So in 2001 the ANTHC—the nation's largest tribal health organization—came up with something called the Dental Health Aide Program. Based upon the principles of the community health aide program, the idea was to identify high school graduates who had grown up in these remote villages and train them to perform basic dental care. They would be people like Kim Baldwin, who already possessed the cultural and linguistic fluency of village life and would, after two years of intense training, return gladly to their hometowns with newfound skills and knowledge. The goal proved harder to accomplish than anyone had ever thought.

—⌘— The Dental Health Aides and Therapists Programs

To begin with, Alaska was starting at ground zero. There was no training program for midlevel dental providers anywhere in the United States. This came as no surprise, since every attempt to introduce such a position had been steadfastly resisted for nearly a century by organized American dentistry. But a 2003 survey by the World Health Organization (WHO) showed that forty-two countries around the world—among them Canada, Great Britain, Australia, and New Zealand—had relied for years on such midlevel providers to educate patients, apply sealants, and perform basic dental procedures, from fillings to extractions, and even root canals.[7]

The Dental Health Therapist Program

This discovery gave the ANTHC the grounds to proceed, and in 2003 it sent the first of three student cohorts—six in each class—to the University of Otago in New Zealand for a two-year training program. Upon graduation, the students would be denominated as "dental health therapists." The ANTHC chose New Zealand because it had more than eighty-five years of experience with this practice model, and Otago is an internationally recognized school of dentistry. The program was funded with a $1 million grant from the Rasmuson Foundation, a private family foundation based in Anchorage devoted to promoting a better life for Alaskans.

The tribal health corporations were underwriting the students' scholarships, and expectations were high. When, in the middle of her first year in New Zealand, Kim Baldwin gave birth to her second daughter, she found herself alone with two small children and a demanding academic workload. Her husband had stayed behind in Alaska to work and support the family. She grew worn out and sick, but felt she couldn't take the time out to see a doctor. She eventually developed strep throat and possibly pneumonia, but pressed on, determined to graduate with her peers. She returned to Alaska to take up practice in January 2006.

The Dental Associations Weigh In

It was almost immediately upon her return that the American Dental Association (ADA) and the Alaska Dental Society (ADS) filed a joint lawsuit in state court against the ANTHC, the state of Alaska, and eight "John Does" (unnamed dental therapists). The dental organizations accused the dental therapists of practicing dentistry without a license, charged the state with failing to enforce the State Dentistry Act, and mounted a no-holds-barred public relations campaign, bombarding the state with ads in newspapers and on radio and TV. One especially arresting ad in the *Juneau Empire* newspaper depicted an openmouthed grizzly bear and bore the caption "Gov. Murkowski—2nd class dental care for Alaska Natives deserves a ferocious reaction!"

In fact, it *was* a ferocious campaign, marshaled to intimidate and distract. The dental organizations lobbied the state's congressional delegation in Washington, D.C., urging them to introduce legislation that would kill the nascent program. They tried to interrupt the state's ability to bill Medicaid for services provided by the new therapists. Hoping to contain any and all midlevel providers to Alaska, they demanded the insertion of specific language in the Indian Health Care Improvement Act to prohibit tribal reservations in the Lower 48 states from using dental therapists. All told, the ADA and the ADS reportedly spent more than $1 million on legal fees, public relations, and lobbyists.[8]

"It was the biggest fight of my life," says Paul Sherry, who spent his teens surfing in Northern California, graduated from Yale University, and in 1974 went to Alaska for a summer as a VISTA volunteer. He never left. In 1976, he married a woman from the village of Minto, northwest of Fairbanks, and twenty-two years later he was the ANTHC's chief executive officer when the lawsuit was filed. In that capacity, he helped lead the group's response. "We didn't expect a lawsuit," he says. "We didn't really have the resources to handle it. We spent half a million dollars to fight it off, and mostly what we had to fight was a public relations campaign." The "public relations campaign" consisted mainly of tribal leaders arguing the merits of the dental therapy program.

If anything, the dental associations' public relations campaign backfired spectacularly. Alaskans took offense at the style and the content of the sledgehammer ad campaign. "It was the condescension more than anything," Sherry says. "The 'we know what's good for you; you don't know what's good for you' attitude." In addition, the dental associations' decision to sue the new, mostly young therapists vexed many in the Native community and struck observers as culturally inept.

"The Inupiat and Yupik cultures are very non-confrontational," says Richard Monkman, the Juneau lawyer who represented the ANTHC. "We felt the only reason they [sued the dental therapists] was to scare these young people. Instead of going back to their communities, they were going to Anchorage giving depositions. The Native community rallied strongly. They saw this as a real attack." Organized dentistry's main argument—that Native people were receiving "second-rate" care—carried little weight among Alaskans who weren't receiving *any* care.

"We objected on constitutional grounds," says Mike Boothe, an Anchorage dentist who helped spearhead the state battle against the therapists. "It was about states' rights. That's why we took on the tribes. The issue of who controls professional licensing—whether in law or medicine—has always been a matter for the states."

"We were defending a legal principle, and legal principles are often difficult to defend," agrees James Towle, executive director of the Alaska Dental Society. "But, yes," he concedes, "we lost the PR battle."

They also lost the lawsuit. In June 2007, Alaskan Superior Court Judge Mark Rindner ruled that dental health therapists were legal under federal statute. The ADA could have filed an appeal but decided to accept the decision—and even paid the ANTHC's legal fees.

To many, it was like a modern-day tale of David and Goliath, a Native nonprofit entity pitted against a powerful lobby bent on resisting any change in the status quo. Medical professionals saw it as a replay of the struggle of nurse practitioners and physician assistants more than forty years earlier.

"They're all the same arguments, and, of course, they all proved inaccurate," says Ruth Ballweg, director of MEDEX Northwest, a University of Washington program that trains physician assistants. "There was a concern that people who weren't doctors couldn't possibly perform primary care procedures such as laceration repair and reduction of simple fractures. In fact, those things are commonly done by nurse practitioners and physician assistants."

There were, however, a few important differences between the two professional bureaucracies that had a role in how the two struggles played out. Doctors have numerous national organizations, especially organizations in their specialty, to choose from besides the American Medical Association; indeed, fewer than 30 percent of all doctors in the United States belong to the AMA. In contrast, the vast majority of dentists are in general practice, and nearly 80 percent of dentists in private practice belong to the American Dental Association. As a result, organized dentistry presents a highly unified and formidable force.

Physicians, furthermore, are accustomed to sharing power from their earliest training in hospitals, where tasks are delegated among a wide array of assistants, including nurses, phlebotomists, and radiologists. That kind of culture does not exist to the same degree in dentistry. "The concept of writing an order and having someone else carry out a task is common in medicine," says Ron Nagel, a dentist who was brought to Alaska in 1999 by the ANTHC to develop a dental aide program. "Not in dentistry. It's protectionism: if they give up those services, they think it erodes their monopoly."

It's easy to dismiss the dentists' concerns as an economic turf war, since dentists rank among the highest paid medical professionals. In Alaska, a first-year dentist can expect to earn $130,000 a year. But the resistance goes deeper. "The American Dental Association wants to promote dentistry as a cottage industry rather than a corporate model," says MEDEX's Ballweg, citing prohibitions in most states against group dental practices and community dental health centers. By going outside individual private practices, the dental therapy movement "brings into question the whole design of how dental care is provided in this country. It's the first crack."

Whatever the reason, the fight in Alaska quickly assumed a negative tone—one that in retrospect prefigured the rancor of the nationwide debate on health care reform in the summer of 2009. Many public health dentists in the state would recount a history of personal vendettas against their careers as a result of their support for dental therapists. Several say their licenses came under scrutiny from the state organization, and many for a time believed their licenses were under threat. Robert Allen, a respected public health dentist in Bethel, was summarily dismissed as secretary of the Alaska Dental Society after declaring at one meeting that dental therapists were "the wave of the future."

The Dental Health Aide Program

From the start, the therapists were intended as part of a larger, tiered program of oral health providers—the goal being to tackle Alaska's oral health crisis on many levels. The first of those levels is the "primary dental health aide I," a position requiring two weeks of training to apply varnishes, give fluoride rinses, and perform patient education. Then there is "primary dental health aide II," with additional responsibilities. At the next level, the "expanded function primary dental health aide" can apply sealants, take X-rays, and perform dental assistance. The highest position is "dental health aide therapist."* According to the original vision,

---

* The hierarchy is somewhat confusing, especially the distinction between *dental health aide therapists,* who have two years of training, and *dental health aides,* who can have as little as two weeks of training. To reduce potential confusion, dental health aide therapists are referred to as *dental therapists* or *dental health therapists* in this chapter.

the aides would act as a kind of "advance guard" of the whole dental armada.

"It's a really critical niche," explains Bornstein, whose 1998 white paper inspired the program. "If we only have dental health therapists filling holes, that wouldn't do the job. That's what dentists have been doing for years—just filling holes. We need to address the bacterial component of the disease. That's what the dental health aides are there for."

In 2004, the Robert Wood Johnson Foundation's Local Initiative Funding Partners program (now called the Local Funding Partnerships program) awarded the ANTHC a two-part grant of $495,000 to train entry-level dental health aides, whose primary focus would be prevention and education. The two weeks of training was to take place in Bethel, a city of roughly 5,500 inhabitants located on the western coast of Alaska. From the beginning, however, there were problems. The dropout rate was high. The pay was low. The ANTHC was distracted by the lawsuit. And the concept itself was questionable. "It was evident that the level of care needed was way beyond the very basic level we were supporting," says Polly Seitz, the director of the Local Funding Partnerships program.

Consequently, when program officers from the Robert Wood Johnson Foundation arrived in Bethel for a site visit in July 2006, they wrote a report critical of the project and expressing unhappiness with the lack of progress. Shortly after, the Foundation decided to rescind the second half of the grant. "The reason the program failed is obvious," says Joel Neimeyer, then a program officer for the Rasmuson Foundation. "You need to address the high levels of oral health disease and intense pain. Afterward, you may want to have a conversation about prevention."

Neimeyer is a civil engineer who worked many years for the U.S. Public Health Service, an independent federal agency, setting up water and sewage facilities around the state. His mother was a Yupik Eskimo from Akiak, a small village on the Kuskokwim River forty miles from Bethel. His father was a Minnesotan of

Norwegian stock; he was a commissioned officer in the Air Force who moved the family every year or two, so that Neimeyer attended four different elementary schools and traveled the world before graduating from high school. As a result, he has always had one foot in both worlds. "I learned a long time ago that even though I did not grow up in Alaska, the culture is within me—my speech patterns, the way I treat people, my sense of humor. I'll be in meetings with folks, the typical graduates from the typical diploma mills around the country, and we'll show up at a meeting and the Native people speak to me." That dual cultural citizenship proved a strong benefit when it came to negotiating between the conflicting interests in the primary dental aide program. Neimeyer says that in hindsight it would have been better to build the dental therapy model before pushing ahead with the primary dental aide model.

Although recently named the federal co-chair of the Denali Commission, Neimeyer maintains an active interest in the dental therapy program. He acknowledges that what happened in Bethel was partly caused by the fact that the program and finance arms of the two different organizations—each separated by more than three hundred miles, with no roads between them—needed to come together at a time when the lawsuit was consuming almost all of the ANTHC's attention.

"Ultimately, it would have been better if the tribal system hadn't got the grant. The ADA was coming down hard, and the ANTHC was in under-siege mentality. All they were trying to do is succeed, and in the middle of it they're bickering because the Robert Wood Johnson Foundation is mad at them. When what they really needed was to be free to focus on the dental therapy program."

Bringing Top Dental Association Officials to Alaska

Neimeyer's boss at the Rasmuson Foundation, Diane Kaplan, the organization's president and chief executive officer, had an idea. She suggested inviting a small group of state and national dental representatives to Alaska so they could see the extent of the oral health problem with their own eyes.

To help cover the expense of the trip, Neimeyer, at Kaplan's recommendation, called David Morse, the vice president for communications at the Robert Wood Johnson Foundation, who approved $15,000 in discretionary funds to cover two trips of local and national dentistry leaders to see the problems firsthand. (The Rasmuson Foundation provided matching funds.) A few weeks later, a contingent of dentists, including Kathleen Roth, then the president of the ADA, flew to Bethel and then by bush plane to the village of Toksook Bay. They attended a *potlatch* in the high school gym, at which tribal elders spoke in Yupik. They met a dental therapist, flew to another village, and met with a local dentist. Subsequently, in a meeting between the ADA team and the health staff in Bethel, one of the ADA officials stated that he realized he wouldn't last more than two days in that frozen environment. To Niemeyer's satisfaction, the visiting dentists *got* it.

The Word Gets Out

By this time, interest in the dental therapy model also was starting to build around the foundation world. "I had some healthy skepticism," acknowledges Albert Yee, a physician who was, at the time, a program director of the W.K. Kellogg Foundation in Battle Creek, Michigan. "I knew that dentists had four years of training after college, and when I saw this program was training high school graduates to do what was then being called 'irreversible procedures,' it raised some eyebrows.

"But then we saw the research. It showed that because they were doing limited scope procedures over and over again they were quite adept at doing those procedures. And as a result, the quality of care by therapists was as good as or better than that of the dentists. That was a bit of an epiphany for us." In mid-2006, the Kellogg Foundation approved an investment of $2.7 million in what would become the DENTEX program.

The DENTEX Program

Because of the great distance to New Zealand, the high cost of training students there, and the desire to find a U.S.-based training site, the ANTHC looked for a training site in the United States. It found one at the University of Washington, which in 1969 had played an important role in the creation of MEDEX Northwest, a pioneering program that trained physician assistants. Now the university was offering to do it again with a program called DENTEX, to replace the one in New Zealand. To the Alaskan and MEDEX leaders alike, it appeared a done deal—until a backlash from dentists affiliated with the Washington State Dental Association led the university's dental school to cancel its participation in the program.

After some last-minute scrambling, the program opened its doors to first-year students in an Anchorage office building a couple of miles from the ANTHC's headquarters. More than 1,400 miles away in Seattle, Louis Fiset, a professor of dentistry, was hired by the University of Washington Medical School to oversee the Alaska program's first-year curriculum and the training of first-year students. (DENTEX provides the curriculum for the second year, but the actual training is done by the ANTHC.) From his perch in the medical school, Fiset developed curriculum, supervised the Anchorage oral health program, evaluated student performance, and coordinated the twenty-three or so dental professors who took turns flying to Alaska from various schools around the United States, teaching one- or two-week modules.

"It was no small thing to put a dental program in the medical school," Ballweg, the director of MEDEX, says. "There were a lot of negotiations behind the scenes, and ultimately the two schools [medical and dental] ended up working together."

In its early days, the program was so controversial that Ballweg and Fiset flat-out refused to identify publicly the dental professors hired to teach the courses, out of fear that they might suffer a backlash. "It just was not safe," Ballweg says. That judgment proved farsighted after a member of the Washington State Dental Association called Ballweg, who is certified as a physician assistant and holds a master's degree in public administration, and demanded that she release the professors' names. "I told her I would not do that. And she said she would ruin my career. Of course, she could not do that. I am not a dentist."

The new DENTEX classroom opened in April 2007, as the first students—all seven of them—arrived at the new Anchorage location for the first in a series of demanding four-week tutorials in anatomy, physiology, infection control, and other subjects. Nominated by their respective tribes, each had received a full scholarship from Alaska's regional health corporations—worth $60,000 a year—to study and, as one Aleutian Islander jokingly put it, "save Alaska one tooth at a time." Students are urged to put their lives on hold for the duration of the two-year program.

Which is just what Bonnie Johnson has done. At nineteen, she shyly allows that she has a good memory and thrives on the challenges posed by the program. But she misses her village of Unalakleet, a close-knit community of about 750 people, many of them related, on the edge of Norton Sound (an inlet of the Bering Sea). Mostly, she misses the traditional foods of home. To keep her spirits up, she has lugged suitcases full of berries, seal oil, dried fish, and dried seal meat, down to Anchorage, enough to last her until her next trip back.

"I grew up in a big, loving family," Johnson says. "I have lots of relatives there. My aunt, Aurora Johnson, was one of the original therapists who went to New Zealand. She told me how difficult the training would be, but she had faith in me."

Today the first-year students are led by clinical site director Mary Willard, an idealistic dentist from Ohio who arrived in Bethel nine years earlier almost on a lark ("I didn't like the cold, but I thought it would look good on my résumé") and fell in love with the town. "There's so much need. You can pick your cause, whatever you want to do. You can be mayor if you want to."

Willard, for her part, took on foster care, providing emergency placement for medically compromised children. One day, while she was on duty at the Bethel hospital, a three-year-old girl was admitted with an oral infection; the right side of her mouth massively swollen. Willard oversaw the girl's medical care, which required intravenous antibiotics and resulted in several teeth being extracted in the operating room. Willard ended up adopting the girl and her two siblings. Today the family lives in Anchorage, where Willard has plans to build the dental therapy program into a national model.

—〰— The Lingering Controversy

A multitude of peer-reviewed studies over the years has shown that dental therapists improve access, help reduce costs, and provide excellent care. In 1992, a double-blind Canadian study found that the quality of tooth restorations by dental therapists was equal to and often better than that of those performed by dentists.[9] A 2007 study by Kenneth Bolin, an assistant professor at Baylor College of Dentistry in Dallas, examined charts from five dental clinics in Alaska and found no statistical difference in the number of complications resulting from treatment delivered by dentists versus therapists.[10] "I've talked with many public health dentists who have supervised the work of therapists, and invariably I've heard the same thing: that the therapists receive more intensive training in their limited scope of work than dentists ever get, and that their skills, when they come out, are better than that of many dentists," says Ron Nagel, the dentist who has been advising the program.

One such therapist is Conan Murat, who maintains a grueling circuit of fourteen villages around the Yukon-Kuskokwim Delta, lugging his portable, back-breakingly heavy operatory (dental chair, air compressor, and equipment) most places he goes. Murat graduated in the first year's class in New Zealand, and he says the school gave him a solid education. But it hardly prepared him for the kind of oral devastation, the "bombed-out teeth," he would routinely see upon his return home. "We really had to adapt when we got back from New Zealand," Murat says. "Like strapping kids into a papoose. I was teaching some new dentists how to do that. They don't practice *that* in dental school. Sometimes parents are crying right in front of you because they realize it's their fault. We're pulling out their kids' teeth and they're crying, 'I'm sorry, I'm sorry.'"

Organized dentistry's opposition to alternative providers has hardly let up. The Patient Protection and Affordable Care Act that was signed into law in March 2010 restricts the dental therapist model to those states where it is already accepted within the scope of practice. But it also funds up to $4 million each for fifteen demonstration sites that will train "alternative dental providers" over a five-year period.

Meanwhile, a groundswell of midlevel providers is gaining traction around the country. In late 2009, a Connecticut State Dental Association task force approved a two-year training program for dental therapists to work in public health settings. The dental association stated that it was not endorsing the model but was willing to study it. Dental delegations from more than a dozen states are now studying workforce issues. One of those is the Washington State Dental Association, which, under new leadership, recently approached Fiset for advice. "Four years ago, they were ready to put a contract out on us," Fiset quips. "Now they're coming to us as the experts."

California, too, is interested. In 2007, the most common reason for emergency room visits in California was for preventable dental conditions—more common than diabetes, according to the California HealthCare Foundation. "I don't think it's going to be as big a battle in California as it was in Alaska," Fiset predicts. "I think the ADA realizes what a disaster befell them [in Alaska]. I don't believe they're going to draw a line in the sand and bring suit against their own kind again. California is too powerful."

Access to oral health care is poised to become part of a larger discussion. Although the national debate on health care reform regularly zeros in on the forty-six million medically uninsured Americans, lack of dental insurance receives less attention. As it happens, for every child without medical insurance, there are at least 2.6 without dental insurance.[11]

These are just statistics. But in February 2007, a twelve-year-old Maryland boy named Deamonte Driver died from an infected tooth for want of simple dental care. His single mother didn't have dental insurance, and few dentists accept Medicaid, with its low reimbursement rates and convoluted bureaucracy. Before Driver's tooth could be extracted, bacteria from the abscess spread to his brain, and the boy died.

That tragedy was cited by Ann Lynch, a Minnesota state senator, as the impetus for choosing dental care as her first issue after getting elected in 2006. She proposed the creation of a new midlevel provider. The response to Lynch's bill resembled the backlash in Alaska. Full page ads attacked Lynch's credibility. Then came a radio campaign and the retention of a public relations company by the Minnesota Dental Association.

In May 2009, Minnesota enacted a law creating a new midlevel provider, but one that fell far short of that in Alaska. In fact, most advocates around the country viewed it as a failure, a concession to organized dentistry. Graduates of the Minnesota program will practice under a more limited scope than their Alaskan counterparts and will be restricted to the direct supervision of a dentist. As a result, advocates charge, they will be relegated to areas of the state where there is in fact no dental shortage.

Perhaps most critical, the legislation prescribes a four-year program. "The kind of student who's attracted to a two-year program is very different from the student who's willing to commit to a four-year program," the Denali Commission's Neimeyer says. "What's going to happen to folks who spend four years going to college in the big city? Are they really going to want to go back home to rural Minnesota?"

In the next few years, such questions will assume new urgency as a pending dentist shortage pushes access to care into the forefront of national attention. A study by the American Dental Education Association predicts a significant shortage of practicing dentists as early as 2014, when more dentists will be retiring than entering the profession.

A sense of urgency has spread throughout the foundation world. At the Robert Wood Johnson Foundation, Denise Davis, a program officer in the health care group, says she has engaged in a series of long conversations with the Kellogg Foundation about the dental therapy program and other possible ways of broadening access to oral care.

"We're interested in reducing disparities in dentistry in a very real way," says Davis, who nonetheless noted that as of September 2010, the Foundation would have no program investment in dentistry. That is when its longstanding investment in the Dental Pipeline program comes to a close. The Foundation has invested $23 million in that program, which encourages dental schools to boost minority admissions and move their clinical rotations outside their institutions and into rural communities.

"These foundations are trying to support each other without getting in each others' way, to think strategically about what they might invest in going forward," says Davis, adding that such cooperation is an unanticipated product of a bad economy. "We are making fewer investments and the investment sizes are smaller," she continues. "So we have to think how best we can leverage what's out there, rather than creating something new."

The future of Alaska's program could well ride on an evaluation of the dental therapist program. The Rasmuson Foundation has committed $526,000 toward it, with Kellogg contributing $1,000,000, and the Bethel Community Services Foundation $93,000. Conducted by RTI International, the evaluation will use independent dental examiners to investigate the quality of the therapists' work, the program's administration, and its ultimate effectiveness.

~~ The Future of Dental Therapists and Dental Aides

The RTI report is expected in October 2010. With a positive result in hand, the ANTHC will be equipped to advance its program. For now, however, the tribal corporation is struggling against an economy of scale. Three years into the program, only twenty dental therapists are working across the state, and Nagel, who retired and moved to Florida in late 2009, estimates that rural Alaska could easily use fifty or sixty therapists.

Meanwhile, the presumptive obituary for primary dental health aides—those assistants trained in prevention, education, and the application of fluoride rinses—may have been premature. In 2008, changes in Medicaid reimbursement allowed providers to charge on an encounter basis. It took a couple of years before administrators and dentists recognized the potential benefit of these new regulations. A primary dental health aide in Alaska can now charge a flat rate of $28.80 for a child's topical fluoride application. As dental clinics around the state become aware of the new rules, there is renewed interest in the training of more aides.

Whether the subject is dental aides or dental therapists, the value of training is partly measured in cost-effectiveness—and Alaska's hard-won expertise could prove a valuable commodity. But until July 2010, as the result of a provision in the settlement of the lawsuit brought by the major dental organizations, the ANTHC was enjoined from promoting its program beyond Alaska's borders. In any event, Alaska's own program still has growing pains. Its administrators struggle with such basic issues as how to identify and recruit strong students, nurture them through the program, and inculcate in them the values of the profession.

In September 2009, twenty-five people responded to the call for applications from the Yukon-Kuskokwim Health Corporation in Bethel, the location of the Robert Wood Johnson Foundation-funded dental aides program. The organization had four dental therapist scholarships to disburse and a hard time giving them away. Many of the initial applicants lost interest once they realized they would be required to move out of their villages for two years of training, according to Troy Wiscombe, manager of the Yukon-Kuskokwim Health Corporation Dental Clinic. Nobody wanted to commit. Two years seemed like a long time, even though the first year's average salary of $60,000 was high by village standards.

In addition, Bethel has had a hard time retaining its dental therapists, leading some administrators to question the investment. As of September 2009, Conan Murat was the only working dental therapist in the region. Technical skills are easier to impart than professional commitment, says Edwin Allgair, a Bethel-based public health dentist who has stood by in frustration as students time and again chose the traditional, subsistence way of life over the demands of career and academics. "'My family's cutting fish right now, I have to go home. It's time for berry picking, my family needs me."

"We can teach the academics, no question about that," Allgair says. "It's attitude and professionalism that we can't teach. That means we have to select for it—identify those student coming into the program beforehand."

Bethel isn't the only hub struggling with these issues, and the reasons are often more complex than first recognized. Stephanie Woods, a dental therapist who half-jokingly calls herself "the queen of extractions," decided to leave her husband's village of Shungnak, population 270, just a couple of years after returning from New Zealand—largely because of its rampant alcoholism. It was everywhere, she says, and she had a child to think about. Today she manages the dental clinic in Kotzebue.

And now, just two years after returning to Kiana, Kim Baldwin and her family have moved to Fairbanks, where life is less expensive and she can give her girls at least one opportunity she never had. "Both my kids want to play piano," she offers in explanation. "I don't play piano. But I think things like that open them up so much."

Baldwin insists she is not quitting her job. She says she loves the work and intends to return to Kiana at least one week out of each month to continue seeing patients. On a recent trip back, she meanders through the village, down to the river to see the fishing haul, and out onto the tundra. Everywhere she goes, she is greeted like a celebrity. "Kim, you're back!"

Notes

1. "Tuberculosis Among American Indians and Alaska Natives—United States, 1985." *Morbidity and Mortality Weekly Report,* August 7, 1987. http://www.cdc.gov/mmwr/preview/mmwrhtml/00000943.htm.
2. Nice P., with Johnson, W. *The Alaska Health Aide Program: A Tradition of Helping Ourselves.* Anchorage: University of Alaska, 1998.
3. U.S. Department of Health and Human Services. *Oral Health in America: A Report of the Surgeon General.* Rockville, Md.: U.S. Department of Health and Human Services, National Institute of Dental and Craniofacial Research, National Institutes of Health, May 2000. http://silk.nih.gov/public/hck1ocv.@www.surgeon.fullrpt.pdf.
4. Edelstein, B. "Dental Care Considerations for Young Children." *Special Care Dentistry,* 2002, *22,* 11S–22S.
5. Indian Health Service. "The 1999 Oral Health Survey of American Indian and Alaskan Native Patients: Findings, Regional Differences and National Comparisons." http://www.dentist.ihs.gov/downloads/Oral_Health_1999_IHS_Survey.pdf.
6. Personal interview with Mark Kelso, D.D.S., Norton Sound Health Corporation, August 2009.
7. World Health Organization. *World Oral Health Country/Area Profile Programme, 2003.* http://www.whocollab.od.mah.se.
8. Personal interview with Kathleen Roth, former president of the ADA, December 2009.
9. Trueblood, G. A. *Quality Evaluation of Specific Dental Services Provided by Canadian Dental Therapists.* Ottawa: Epidemiology and Community Health Specialties, Health and Welfare Canada, 1992.
10. Bolin, K. "Assessment of Treatment Provided by Dental Health Aide Therapists in Alaska: A Pilot Study." *Journal of the American Dental Association,* 2008, *139,* 1530–1535.
11. Centers for Disease Control and Prevention. "Children's Oral Health." 2004. http://www.cdc.gov/oralhealth/publications/factsheets/sgr2000_fs3.htm

Section Three
Combating Substance Abuse

The Substance Abuse Policy Research Program

David G. Altman, Marjorie A. Gutman, Prabhu Ponkshe,
Andrea Williams, and Susan Frye

Editors' Introduction

In volume XII of the *Anthology,* James Marks, senior vice president of the
Robert Wood Johnson Foundation, and Joseph Alper, an award-winning health
care journalist, wrote, "While direct services grants can improve the health of
individuals and communities, foundation support for changes in public policy
has the potential to reach far greater numbers of people and create lasting
improvements."[1] To provide policy solutions to problems, the Robert Wood
Johnson Foundation has developed a unique set of research programs whose
strength is to provide the evidence for solutions that will stick long after the
Foundation's programming ends. In some cases, the Foundation has fortified
the research by funding communications and advocacy efforts to promote policy
changes.

　　　　　The best example comes from the Foundation's work on tobacco. The
Substance Abuse Policy Research Program and its predecessor, the Tobacco
Policy Research and Evaluation Program, developed evidence of effective policy

interventions, including tobacco taxes, public funding of cessation efforts, and clean indoor air laws. The Center for Tobacco-Free Kids provided strategic communications that advanced the evidence-based policy interventions. In forty-eight states, coalitions supported by the SmokeLess States program advocated changes in state policies and regulations that were based on the evidence provided by Foundation-funded policy research. Finally, the Foundation funded two programs, Bridging the Gap and Monitoring the Future, to assess the results of its tobacco-control efforts.

In this chapter, leaders of the Substance Abuse Policy Research Program look back at the program, which ended in 2009, and reflect on how the program operated and on what its policy research on tobacco, alcohol, and drugs accomplished. David Altman, executive vice president of the Center for Creative Leadership, was the program's director; Marjorie Gutman, currently president of Gutman Research Associates, was the co-director; Prabhu Ponkshe, president of Health Matrix, Inc., served as communications director; Andrea Williams and Susan Frye, both of whom are based at the Center for Creative Leadership, served as the deputy director and grants administrator, respectively.

The Foundation has applied the model of evidence-based research pioneered by the Substance Abuse Policy Research Program to its childhood obesity work. The Healthy Eating Research program, which the Foundation has funded since 2005, is designed to develop research around environmental and policy interventions to promote eating of more nutritious foods. The Active Living Research program supports research on environmental and policy influences on childhood obesity. Both programs follow the Substance Abuse Policy Research Program model of including communications efforts to bring research findings to the attention of policy makers.

Note

1. Marks, J. S., and Alper, J. "Shaping Public Policy as a Robert Wood Johnson Foundation Approach." *To Improve Health and Health Care, Vol. XII: The Robert Wood Johnson Foundation Anthology.* San Francisco: Jossey-Bass, 2009, p. 95.

—ᨙ— U ntil the last decade of the twentieth century, neither the federal government nor foundations considered tobacco policy research worthy of being named as a priority, and only a handful of researchers focused on tobacco policy. That changed in 1991, when the Robert Wood Johnson Foundation made lowering young peoples' use of tobacco one of its priorities. Tobacco control was one element of the Foundation's goal to reduce the harm caused by substance abuse. To reach that goal, the Foundation pursued a three-part strategy: generating a knowledge base, demonstrating and evaluating solutions, and building capacity and momentum for policy change.

In 1992, the Foundation allocated $5 million to fund the Tobacco Policy Research and Evaluation Program, whose goal was to support multidisciplinary research on all aspects of tobacco policy. Midway through the program, the Foundation decided to expand its commitment to policy research, and in 1994 it authorized $12 million to establish the Substance Abuse Policy Research Program, which supported research on alcohol and drug policy as well as tobacco policy. Over roughly fifteen years (funding for the research grants ended in 2009, and funding for the national program office at the Center for Creative Leadership in Greensboro, North Carolina, ended in early-2010), the Foundation authorized $66 million for the Substance Abuse Policy Research Program, which in turn awarded nearly 370 grants to enable researchers to conduct investigations in this new field.[1]

—ᨙ— The Substance Abuse Policy Research Program: Organization and Development

The primary goals of the Substance Abuse Policy Research Program were to support policy-relevant research projects on ways to reduce the harm caused by tobacco, alcohol, and drugs; create a field of substance abuse policy research by supporting senior investigators and attracting new researchers; and disseminate knowledge generated by the research to journalists, researchers, policy makers, and advocacy organizations. The program also sought to nurture the field by leveraging additional support for policy research.

Organizational Structure

Located initially at the Wake Forest University School of Medicine and later at the Center for Creative Leadership, the national program office has remained relatively small. Originally consisting only of a part-time director and deputy director, the program, recognizing the importance of disseminating research reports, expanded to include a part-time director of communications.

The most important task of the program was to support policy-relevant, peer-reviewed research. To help it select among competing research proposals, the national program office recruited a broad and diverse pool of reviewers. (The national program office maintained a database of five hundred reviewers.) To provide expertise on the issues, to help guide the process of developing a research agenda, and to infuse a policy perspective into the review process, the national program office recruited senior program consultants. Initially, there were three such consultants, one for each major substance abuse area (tobacco, alcohol, and drugs). Additional consultants were added during the life of the program. By its close, nine senior consultants had helped to guide the program.

Grantmaking Under the Substance Abuse Research Program

Between 1995 and 2009, grants made by the Substance Abuse Policy Research Program funded studies that focused on policies related to alcohol (14 percent), tobacco (32 percent), and other drugs (23 percent). Nearly one-third of the funding (31 percent) was for multisubstance studies, mostly focusing on alcohol and drugs.

Over its history, the Substance Abuse Policy Research Program made four kinds of awards:

- Grants of $100,000 to $400,000 were made to applicants submitting proposals in response to calls for proposals. The once- or twice-yearly calls for proposals ranged from fairly open to highly targeted solicitations. Overall, the Substance Abuse Policy Research Program sought to fund those proposals of the greatest scientific quality and with the greatest potential for policy impact.

- Grants of less than $100,000 were awarded on an expedited basis in response to a proposal submitted by investigators. This type of grant was designed for rapid deployment, such as when a policy was unexpectedly being put into place, and it was important to collect baseline data quickly. As the program unfolded, it became evident that these smaller grants worked well for studies employing secondary analysis of large data sets and for newer investigators. Some of the most productive and groundbreaking studies were supported with small grants.

- Targeted Rapid Response Grants—small grants, usually less than $50,000, related to a specific and time-sensitive issue—were typically awarded to a partnership between a frontline organization and a researcher. These targeted grants were generally used to increase the capacity of state and local government entities to conduct useful, timely policy analysis and apply it to policy. This mechanism was later adopted by other Robert Wood Johnson Foundation-funded research programs.

- Diversity Partnership Grants allowed minority investigators to apply for a grant of up to $40,000 a year for three years to conduct a study that supplemented an existing Substance Abuse Policy Research Program study. This approach was adopted by the Robert Wood

Johnson Foundation's New Connections program
and by other research programs to encourage diversity
among health researchers.

As of July 2010, more than $140 million in research funding
via two hundred spin-off grants had been awarded to Substance
Abuse Policy Research Program investigators subsequent to their
having received funding from the program. In other words, each
dollar invested in an investigator generated more than $2 of
additional research funding from other sources.

Communications and Dissemination

Publishing scientific findings remains the key to establishing
the scientific credibility of the Substance Abuse Policy Research
Program–funded research, particularly if results are published in
peer-reviewed scientific journals. Since the program's inception
in 1994, more than two hundred peer-reviewed journals across
disciplines published research supported by the program.

To ensure the program's research results got wider visibility,
the national program office developed a strategic communications
effort. It included a Web site, media and congressional briefings,
press releases, print or broadcast stories in the thousands, articles in
substance abuse trade and professional publications, and regular
interaction with policy makers and journalists. The program
published a newsletter, *Addiction Policy Research Update*, that was
distributed widely to policy makers, journalists, advocacy groups,
and researchers. It is available on the Substance Abuse Policy
Research Program's Web site, along with twenty-four *Knowledge
Assets*, distillations of knowledge produced for the Web site.

In addition, the program collaborated with the Addiction
Studies Program, funded by the National Institute on Drug
Abuse and run through the Wake Forest University School of
Medicine, to link journalists and policy makers to the Substance
Abuse Policy Research Program's research.

—⁓— Substance Abuse Policy Research and Its Impact

Over the years, many of the 370 projects that the Substance Abuse Policy Research Program funded have contributed to the overall debate on substance abuse policies. Researchers have given briefings to policy and advocacy groups, participated in news conferences, testified before legislative committees, filed court briefings (including briefings with the United States Supreme Court), and served as expert witnesses in court proceedings.

The Substance Abuse Policy Research Program has developed a framework for categorizing the research it has funded. Rather than use categories such as tobacco, alcohol, and drugs, it has considered how the research has informed the policy process. The end points of informing the policy process with scientific information are as follows:

1. Answering issues of concern to policy makers

2. Raising entirely new questions that policy makers have not asked and then providing the answers to those questions

3. Softening the ideological rhetoric with evidence

4. Developing game changers and tipping points

A few case studies within each of these categories will illustrate the kinds of policy research funded by the program and the impact that some of the research has had.

Answering Issues of Concern to Policy Makers

The Substance Abuse Policy Research Program has been able to respond to requests from policy makers for research on a variety of approaches to reducing substance abuse. Two significant examples are the research conducted to determine whether the Synar Amendment was reducing sales of cigarettes to minors and to investigate the effectiveness of alcohol ignition interlocking devices on drunk driving. Each of these is discussed below.

Enforcement of the Synar Amendment Prohibiting Tobacco Sales to Minors

In 1992, Congress enacted the Synar Amendment, which required states and territories to enact laws prohibiting the sale of tobacco to minors and to enforce them in a manner that could reasonably be expected to decrease the availability of tobacco to minors. The Department of Health and Human Services (DHHS) was ordered to withhold block grant funding from noncompliant states.

A few years after the law had passed, policy makers wanted to know whether the Synar Amendment had achieved its purpose. The Substance Abuse Policy Research Program funded University of Massachusetts Medical School researcher Joseph DiFranza's examination of whether states had enacted a tobacco sales law, conducted enforcement inspections, penalized violators, and conducted a statewide survey. The study also examined whether DHHS regulations and actions were consistent with the statutory requirements of the Synar Amendment.

DiFranza found in 1997 that both the states and DHHS were violating the statutory requirements of the Synar Amendment, rendering it ineffective. Few states had implemented effective enforcement programs, and national surveys confirmed that there had been no measurable reduction in the availability of tobacco to young people. These results served notice to the states and to the federal government that their implementation of the Synar Amendment was being scrutinized by independent researchers.

In subsequent studies conducted between 1997 and 2003, DiFranza found similar results.[2] He also found that as implementation and enforcement of the Synar Amendment increased, cigarette sales decreased.[3] DiFranza's studies demonstrated that research can be used to provide oversight on the implementation of policies and in evaluating the impact of a policy on behavior.

Alcohol Ignition Interlocking Devices

To address the public safety risks posed by habitual drunk drivers, the Colorado General Assembly authorized a voluntary alcohol ignition interlock pilot program in 1995.[4] An alcohol ignition interlock is an electronic device that is mounted on a vehicle's dashboard and connected to its ignition system. The driver is required to blow into the device; if the driver's blood alcohol level is above a specified level, the vehicle cannot be started. Interlocks also require "rolling retests" while the car is in motion. In 1999, four years after the original legislation, a law was passed requiring that interlocks be installed on cars driven by individuals with two or more alcohol offenses within a five-year period and that the interlock be used for a period of one year after license reinstatement.

The Substance Abuse Policy Research Program funded University of Colorado Health Science Center researcher William Marine to determine whether the interlock program had enrolled high-risk repeat offenders and whether interlock use reduced repeat drunk driving offenses. Marine's research, co-funded by the state of Colorado in response to emerging interest in policies on interlock devices, found that the voluntary interlock program had enrolled nine hundred DUI offenders in its first three years. Although this was an important achievement, it represented a very small fraction of the more than thirty-seven thousand Colorado motorists arrested for DUI in 1998 alone.

Marine also found that offenders who installed interlocks had a lower rate of rearrest for alcohol-related offenses than individuals who had not applied for or installed interlock devices.[5] In part because of the Substance Abuse Policy Research Program–funded research, the Colorado legislature required repeat alcohol offenders after 2001 to have an ignition interlock installed on their vehicles before their driving privileges were reinstated. Reinstated licenses were restricted to the use of vehicles equipped with an approved ignition interlock.

Raising New Questions and Providing the Answers

Substance abuse policy research is as much about raising new questions and providing answers to them as it is about answering questions that are already being asked. Two illustrations of research proposed by investigators looking at new issues are office-based methadone treatment and drugged driving.

Office-Based Methadone Treatment

Methadone has been used in the treatment of heroin addiction for more than fifty years and has been found to be effective in reducing drug use, improving social behavior and personal productivity, and preventing the spread of infectious diseases. Traditionally, all recovering heroin addicts have had to get their methadone every day from specialized treatment centers. The treatment centers are highly regulated and are difficult to establish and maintain. Almost two hundred thousand patients receive treatment at these specialized centers, but many more people need methadone than the treatment centers can serve.

The questions raised by the Substance Abuse Policy Research Program grantee Joseph Merrill of the University of Washington and Harborview Medical Center in Seattle were: Is it possible to transfer some patients from community treatment programs to primary care facilities, thereby creating space for those waiting to get methadone from the centers? And how difficult is it for a primary care facility to get the necessary legal clearances to provide methadone treatment?

Merrill found that providing methadone treatment in a primary care setting was feasible and could result in healthy outcomes for patients addicted to heroin who were stable on methadone.[6] The primary care setting requires fewer treatment visits and allows patients to take more of their medication at home. His studies also found that primary care facilities can be successful in helping patients address their heroin addiction effectively while providing treatment for other health problems and improving physician attitudes about addiction.[7]

The study found that getting the necessary state and local regulatory approvals to provide methadone in a primary care setting could be difficult, but it also indicated how the regulatory processes could be navigated.

Drugged Driving

Each year, millions of Americans reportedly drive shortly after using marijuana or cocaine. Why is it difficult to identify, prosecute, or treat drugged drivers? That question was posed by the Substance Abuse Policy Research Program grantee J. Michael Walsh, president of The Walsh Group. Walsh is a former executive director of the President's Drug Advisory Council.

The answer, Walsh discovered, was that there are no national standards for testing drugged drivers, and too few police officers are trained to detect drivers who may be under the influence of drugs. In 2002, Walsh wrote a report on drugged driving that was published in collaboration with the American Bar Association's Standing Committee on Substance Abuse. The report, which was informed by experts in fields such as substance use, traffic safety, auto insurance, and law enforcement, found that laws affecting driving under the influence of drugs fell into three main categories. Some states required that the drugs render a driver incapable of safely operating a vehicle. Other states required that the drug "impair" the driver's ability to operate a vehicle safely or required the driver to be "under the influence of or affected by an intoxicating drug." A small group of states had zero tolerance (or *per se*) laws, which make it a criminal offense to have a drug or metabolite in the body while operating a motor vehicle.[8]

Walsh found that the first two types of laws, which were in existence in forty-two states, made it extremely difficult for prosecutors to prove that the incapacity or impairment of the driver was directly related to the drug ingested. The zero tolerance laws found in eight states at the time made it easier to prosecute a drugged driving charge. Walsh's study has been the basis of several subsequent reports, and according to an opinion piece by Walsh published in *The Washington Post* in 2007, fifteen states had passed legislation establishing *per se* standards.[9]

Softening the Ideological Rhetoric

The policy debates around substance abuse often touch on other social issues, such as poverty, race, housing, and welfare. There is also some stigma associated with individuals who are dependent on drugs and alcohol—individuals who are not politically powerful. These conditions create a significant amount of ideological rhetoric in the policy debates surrounding prevention and treatment for drug and alcohol abuse. Research-based evidence has had a softening effect on some of these sharp policy debates.

Crack Babies

Crack cocaine use, which took society by surprise in the 1980s, quickly became an epidemic. A particularly polarizing issue was the use of crack cocaine by pregnant women. Early reports linked prenatal cocaine exposure to physical and mental damage to the child and resulted in a rush to judgment that these children were beyond hope and destined to become wards of society (and that draconian penalties were appropriate for the mothers).

To provide a rational, science-based perspective, from 1996 to 1999 the Substance Abuse Policy Research Program funded Barry Lester of Brown University to develop a computerized database containing all of the published studies on prenatal cocaine exposure and child outcomes. After analyzing the information in the database, Lester was able to demonstrate that of the more than one hundred published studies, only five had followed cocaine-exposed children through school age. Lester's study showed that the effects of cocaine use by mothers on their children were mild and subtle and that these effects were not observed among all children.[10]

The review also showed, however, that even subtle effects affect a large number of children and require additional resources from society. The evidence did not indicate that these children suffered irreparable damage. Through prevention and intervention programs, it was possible to identify the children who needed help and to provide services to facilitate their normal development.

Lester's work put the problem within the context of environmental factors such as poverty, stress, violence, and poor parenting—factors that can affect a child even without drugs. Because of these factors, it was difficult but not impossible to tease out the effects of cocaine exposure *in utero*. His research was cited in several court cases challenging the validity of sanctions against women who used cocaine during pregnancy.

Homeless Alcoholics

Significant amounts of taxpayers' dollars in every major city go toward police and emergency health care services that are provided for the homeless, and especially for homeless alcoholics. In 1997, a decision by the Downtown Emergency Service Center, a nonprofit organization in King County (Seattle), Washington, to provide housing and support services for homeless alcoholics resulted in a sharp political debate. Many policy makers, ordinary citizens, and business interests argued in favor of leaving homeless alcoholics on the street rather than providing them with services that would siphon money from other needed services.

This debate nearly ended, at least in Seattle, after the Substance Abuse Policy Research Program grantee Mary Larimer of the University of Washington found that the initiative, called Housing First, saved taxpayers more than $4 million dollars in the first year of operation. During the first six months, even after considering the cost of administering housing for the ninety-five residents in a

Housing First program in downtown Seattle, the study reported an average cost savings of 53 percent—nearly $2,500 a month per person in health and social services—compared with a control group of homeless alcoholics.[11]

The study found that stable housing also reduced drinking among homeless alcoholics, even though Housing First did not require participants to stop drinking. The longer the alcoholics stayed in the program, the less they drank, according to the study, which has generated interest from many other cities around the country. Larimer and her co-authors noted, "In most U.S. cities, people with behavioral health disabilities die on the streets far more frequently than any other subset of the homeless population. Before they die, they use large amounts of taxpayer-funded services in the healthcare and criminal justice systems. The King County housing program was created to stabilize people and stop them from endlessly cycling through emergency rooms, prisons and other crisis institutions, reducing the amount of taxpayer money spent on them."[12]

Developing Game Changers

The last category, "game changers," shows that rigorous policy research by several independent researchers examining an issue from multiple perspectives can stimulate significant shifts in policy.

Tobacco Taxes

During the 1980s, the idea of raising state or federal excise taxes on tobacco products drew much criticism as an unsound economic policy that unfairly penalized a legitimate industry and its loyal customers. Fast-forward to 2009, when there was a sense of inevitability and only muted opposition to a 61-cent federal tax increase on a pack of cigarettes to pay for a children's health insurance initiative. Also, by the end of 2009, the average cigarette tax across all states was $1.34 a pack, with forty-six states, the

District of Columbia, and several United States territories having increased their cigarette tax rates more than ninety-five times between 2002 and 2009.

The overwhelming evidence of the harmful consequences of smoking, although critical, would probably not by itself have resulted in as much change as actually occurred. The many studies, some of them funded by the Substance Abuse Policy Research Program, demonstrating that increasing tobacco taxes both reduced smoking among vulnerable groups and raised revenues, created the traction for a national and grassroots advocacy movement led by the Campaign for Tobacco-Free Kids. The combination of policy research and advocacy changed the policy debate around tobacco taxes.

Over the years, the Substance Abuse Policy Research Program supported thirty-three studies on tobacco taxes and pricing, resulting in ninety-seven publications. One of the first studies began in 1993 under a grant from the Tobacco Policy Research and Evaluation Program (predecessor to the Substance Abuse Policy Research Program) and was conducted by Frank Chaloupka at the University of Illinois at Chicago. That study found that smoking among youth was about three times as sensitive to price as smoking among adults; it estimated that a 10 percent price increase would reduce the prevalence of youth smoking by nearly 7 percent.[13] Subsequent research by Substance Abuse Policy Research Program grantees and others has contributed to the overwhelming evidence today that tobacco taxes are an effective way of reducing tobacco consumption.

Federal Regulation of Nicotine as a Drug

In the early 1990s, the idea that nicotine met the Food and Drug Administration's definition of a drug and thus should come under its regulatory authority was discussed in Washington policy circles. In 1993, the Substance Abuse Policy Research Program funded an unusual study by John Slade of St. Peters Medical Center and the University of Medicine and Dentistry of New Jersey.

Slade conducted a detailed analysis of the documents generated by and about the tobacco industry—court documents, patents, scientific papers generated by industry-supported scientists, industry newsletters, and other public documents—to determine whether nicotine fit the legal definition of a drug. Slade's extensive research led him to conclude that nicotine fit the legal definition of a drug.

In 1995, the FDA proposed regulating nicotine as a drug and cigarettes as a device that delivers nicotine to the body. Slade used his research to provide a formal commentary on the proposed regulations on behalf of the American Society for Addiction Medicine. It was the second most extensive commentary submitted, exceeded only by that from the tobacco industry. In its final ruling in 1996, the FDA cited Slade's commentary several times, as well as other studies funded by the Substance Abuse Policy Research Program's precursor, the Tobacco Policy Research and Evaluation Program.

Even though the United States Supreme Court blocked the FDA from regulating tobacco in 2000, Slade's analysis contributed to defining the problem and making it more visible. Advocates and the media picked up and publicized the information from Slade's commentary demonstrating that the tobacco industry had deceived the American public about the addictive nature and harmful effects of nicotine, the key ingredient in tobacco. This helped to cement the public's view that the tobacco industry was deceitful and that regulation of tobacco products was necessary. In 2009, Congress passed legislation empowering the FDA to regulate nicotine as a drug.

—⁓— Communicating Research Findings

In 2005, White Mountain Research Associates did an assessment of the information needs of the Substance Abuse Policy Research Program's policy audiences. The findings revealed that policy makers need reliable information presented in a concise format. Policy makers found research data and statistics from the Substance Abuse Policy Research Program highly credible, but they preferred the information in a more accessible format. They reported wanting "bulleted lists" and "bite-size" conclusions. They also wanted to be able to access this information online.

Knowledge Assets

The Substance Abuse Policy Research Program's *Knowledge Assets* were developed to address these needs. Each *Knowledge Asset* is written by a leading researcher and reviewed by a team of independent researchers; each summarizes a comprehensive body of information focused on a particular substance abuse issue. The *Knowledge Assets* format includes an overview of the topic, implications for policy, and research results from the Substance Abuse Policy Research Program–funded studies and other studies. The overview, implications, and key results average only one and a half pages and can be compiled into a printable policy brief. Each *Knowledge Asset* also includes links to more detailed research results and other resources, allowing users to delve more deeply into a topic of interest.

As of July 2010, the Substance Abuse Policy Research Program had published twenty-four *Knowledge Assets* (see Exhibit 7.1). The program has disseminated Knowledge Assets widely to policy makers, journalists, and researchers. Traffic to the program's Web site triples as new *Knowledge Assets* are released.

Social Networking Activities

In the fall of 2009, the Substance Abuse Policy Research Program began testing a number of social networking strategies to leverage the Robert Wood Johnson Foundation's investment in

Exhibit 7.1.   Knowledge Assets Published Through July 2010

Topic Area	Knowledge Asset Title	Authors
Alcohol	"Binge Drinking on College Campuses and in Communities"	Traci L. Toomey, Ph.D., Toben F. Nelson, Sc.D., and Kathleen Lenk, M.P.H., School of Public Health, University of Minnesota
Alcohol	"Alcohol Retail Policy"	Traci L. Toomey, Ph.D., School of Public Health, University of Minnesota
Alcohol	"American Indian and Alaska Native Alcohol Policies"	Paul Spicer, Ph.D., Center for Applied Social Research, University of Oklahoma
Alcohol	"DUI Policy"	Alexander C. Wagenaar, Ph.D., and Amy L. Tobler, M.P.H., University of Florida, College of Medicine, Department of Epidemiology and Health Policy Research
Alcohol	"Minimum Legal Drinking Age Policy"	James C. Fell, M.S., Pacific Institute for Research and Evaluation
Drugs	"Buprenorphine Treatment for Opioid Addiction"	Robin E. Clark, Ph.D., and Jeffrey D. Baxter, M.D., Center for Health Policy and Research and Department of Family Medicine and Community Health, University of Massachusetts Medical School
Drugs	"Drug Testing of Adolescents in Schools"	Sharon Levy, M.D., M.P.H., Harvard Medical School
Drugs	"Drug Treatment for Drug-Abusing Criminal Offenders: Insights from California's Proposition 36 and Arizona's Proposition 200"	Beau Kilmer, Ph.D., RAND Drug Policy Research Center, and Martin Y. Iguchi, Ph.D., UCLA School of Public Health, Department of Community Health Sciences
Drugs	"Syringe Access Interventions"	Scott Burris, J.D., Beasley School of Law, Temple University
Drugs	"Treating Opioid Addiction in an Office-Based Practice"	Joseph Merrill, M.D., M.P.H., Division of General Internal Medicine, Harborview Medical Center
Multisubstance	"Substance Abuse and Healthcare Costs"	Robin E. Clark, Ph.D., Elizabeth O'Connell, M.S., and Mihail Samnaliev, Ph.D., Center for Health Policy and Research and Department of Family Medicine and Community Health, University of Massachusetts Medical School

Exhibit 7.1. (*Continued*)

Topic Area	Knowledge Asset Title	Authors
Multisubstance	"Barriers to Treating Alcohol and Drug Problems Among Adolescents"	Hannah K. Knudsen, Ph.D., Department of Behavioral Science and Center on Drug and Alcohol Research, University of Kentucky
Multisubstance	"Co-occurring Disorders"	Mark McGovern, Dartmouth Medical School
Multisubstance	"Cost-Effectiveness of Substance Abuse Treatment in Criminal Justice Settings"	Kathryn McCollister, Ph.D., Miller School of Medicine, University of Miami
Multisubstance	"Racial and Ethnic Disparities in Substance Abuse Treatment"	Laura A. Schmidt, Ph.D., M.S.W., M.P.H., Philip R. Lee Institute for Health Policy Studies, University of California at San Francisco, and Nina Mulia, Dr.P.H., Alcohol Research Group, Public Health Institute
Multisubstance	"Substance Abuse and Welfare Reform"	Lisa Metsch, Ph.D., University of Miami School of Medicine, and Harold Pollack, Ph.D., School of Social Service Administration, University of Chicago
Multisubstance	"Substance Abuse Treatment Benefits and Costs"	Dennis McCarty, Ph.D., Oregon Health and Science University
Tobacco	"Cigarette Taxes and Pricing"	Frank Chaloupka, Ph.D., Institute for Health Research and Policy, University of Illinois at Chicago
Tobacco	"Clean Indoor Air"	Andrew Hyland, Ph.D., Health Research, Inc., Roswell Park Cancer Institute
Tobacco	"Increasing the Use of Smoking Cessation Treatments"	K. Michael Cummings, Ph.D., Department of Health Behavior, Roswell Park Cancer Institute
Tobacco	"Internet Cigarette Sales"	Kurt M. Ribisl, Ph.D., and Rebecca S. Williams, M.H.S., Ph.D., School of Public Health, University of North Carolina at Chapel Hill; Annice E. Kim, M.P.H., Ph.D., Research Triangle Institute

the program. The program plans to use social networking tools to achieve the following aims:

1. Transfer the vast substance abuse policy research knowledge base to the public domain

2. Recruit and mobilize experts to encourage discussion as it pertains to the knowledge base

3. Conduct a scientific experiment using social networking to examine the impact on dissemination

4. Inform policy makers, journalists, researchers, advocates, and the public about substance abuse policy research and findings

5. Connect researchers around substance abuse policy research

As a limited first step, the program implemented some selected social media and networking strategies (blogs, Twitter, YouTube) to disseminate knowledge generated by researchers during congressional briefings. The YouTube videos, which are already available, have generated additional conversations among researchers and between researchers and lay audiences.

—⟋⟍— Future Investment and Direction

With the Substance Abuse Policy Research Program having closed in 2009, three areas of future investment for substance abuse policy research are still needed: funding for policy research; other kinds of resources to support the field; and strategic communication of findings to inform policy.

Funding for Policy Research

The field of substance abuse policy research will continue to need funding for new studies. Although some funding is available through federal research institutes and state agencies, there is no indication any of these entities will expand its funding sufficiently to replace the contribution of the Robert Wood Johnson Foundation. Yet policy needs keep increasing and requiring new studies. Responding to this, the Substance Abuse Policy Research Program conducted a yearlong effort involving several dozen investigators and other stakeholders to develop a set of research agendas, or blueprints, for the field over the next five years.[14]

Resources to Support Investigators and the Field

Efforts are still needed to attract young investigators and provide them with opportunities for networking, sharing ideas, and building skills. Young investigators reinforce the Substance Abuse Policy Research Program experience when they report that smaller and supplemental grants provided excellent opportunities for them to win grants from non-program funding sources and jump-start their careers.[15] Conferences, invitational meetings, Webinars, and Internet professional networks provide opportunities to continue and expand networking among investigators from various disciplines who have a common interest in these areas of policy research.

Communicating Policy Research

The need to communicate research findings to policy makers will probably grow in the future. Policy makers and advocates, the media, and investigators will continue to need the resources the Substance Abuse Policy Research Program Web site offers, including links to publications and Knowledge Assets.

—∿— Lessons from the Substance Abuse Policy Research Program

The Substance Abuse Policy Research Program's work for more than fifteen years has led to several lessons about policy-relevant research, growing a nascent field, and making research findings useful for policy makers.

Policy Impact Requires a Long-Term View

Investment in policy research generally needs to be of several years' duration. This allows evidence to accumulate across individual studies, eventually yielding products that synthesize a body of evidence for major topics and that can be widely shared through vehicles such as policy briefs, Knowledge Assets, and systematic scientific reviews. One study, or even several studies, rarely yields sufficient evidence to credibly guide policy. A multiyear initiative allows the research and the policy communities to interact over a period of time. New evidence can be brought to bear on the policy process, informing the development of new policies, which can, in turn, engender further research to assess their feasibility, effectiveness, and consequences. Longer-term funding also permits a program to become a more visible and credible source of information for researchers, the media, policy makers, and advocates.

It Is Important to Support Innovative Research and Take Risks

The Substance Abuse Policy Research Program experience suggests that promoting innovation, experimenting, and taking risks can pay off. Provided the science was strong and the potential for policy relevance was high, the Substance Abuse Policy Research Program regularly funded studies that were innovative. For example, at the time the study on ignition interlock devices was being considered, the devices were being pilot tested as a policy tool to reduce drunk driving. Ignition interlock devices have become an increasingly well-known and tested part of the criminal justice response to drinking and driving. Another example is the Substance Abuse Policy Research Program's grant to a partnership between a university and a human services organization in Seattle to study the effectiveness of Housing First, an approach that provides housing to homeless individuals with alcohol dependence without requiring that they first become abstinent. None of the members of the review committee had heard of the Housing First approach but thought it merited a rigorous test. Since the positive results of that study were published, additional locales have adopted the approach.

The program's efforts to attract principal investigators from underrepresented groups also broke new ground. The goal of nurturing the careers of individuals from minority groups was not new, but specific components used by the Substance Abuse Policy Research Program, such as adding supplemental grants for minority researchers to existing research projects, had not been tried previously. This model has since been adapted by other Robert Wood Johnson Foundation–funded national research programs.

Another aspect of promoting innovation was incorporating technological advances into the program, such as development of a relational, searchable program database, and social networking experiments conducted in the Web 2.0 environment.

Sustaining Program Elements Is Challenging but Critical

The Substance Abuse Policy Research Program had mixed results in sustaining its work:

- Stimulating and facilitating investigators to leverage additional funding was a productive strategy, yielding approximately two dollars for every dollar awarded by the program.

- Obtaining additional and sustainable funding for the program was less successful. Although the program's staff members had solid relationships with other funding agencies, a number of barriers affected the willingness of these organizations to supplement or replace the Robert Wood Johnson Foundation's funding. Substance abuse tends to lack appeal for private foundations because of general stigma; private foundations do not generally fund research; the overwhelming majority of federal research agency or institute funding is devoted to biomedical and clinical research; and some policy research is just too controversial for government funding organizations to take on. Concerted efforts to enlist other funding organizations need to occur in the early years of a program. Early establishment of a partnership or collaborative with other funding organizations, particularly one offering pooled funding (such as the National Collaborative on Childhood Obesity Research, which is supported by the Centers for Disease Control and Prevention, National Institutes of Health, and Department of Agriculture) might have created a viable strategy for sustaining funding.

Communications Are a Key to Making Research Relevant to Policy Makers and the Public

The Substance Abuse Policy Research Program experience provides several lessons regarding strategic communications of research findings, including the following:

- Making communications a priority and developing an independent communications effort can enhance the capacity for using evidence from research to inform policy debates. To make communications a priority, the Substance Abuse Policy Research Program hired a communications director, developed a strategic communications plan, and devoted funds to communications activities.

- The communications effort is inseparable from the scientific aspects of the program. The communications director worked closely with the rest of the national program office leadership. In this way, the research is respected and conveyed accurately, and both investigators and the program's scientific leadership gained skills and comfort as active, savvy partners in the communications effort.

- A multifaceted strategic communications campaign that uses multiple approaches (for example, directly to policy makers, to the media, to advocates) and methods (such as editorials, media briefings, and congressional briefings) is needed.

- Triaging is essential to strategic communications. The communications director, in collaboration with the program's director and co-director, continually assessed which studies were getting ready to publish findings and which findings were most pertinent to current policy debates and then allocated communications resources accordingly.

⎯⎯ Conclusion

As a midcourse evaluation of the program conducted by The Lewin Group in 1999 concluded, "The Substance Abuse Policy Research Program and its funded research are succeeding in building the field of substance abuse policy research and have influenced the focus of the debate in this area."[16] More specifically, the evaluation found that the program enhanced the careers of both early and established investigators and attracted researchers from other disciplines to enter the field of substance abuse policy research.

Investigators funded by the program represented a wide array of disciplines, including anthropology, psychology, economics, sociology, public health, medicine, history, and political science. About 20 percent of the investigators who received funding reported being in the early stages of their careers, and more than two-thirds had not received previous funding related to substance abuse policy research. At the same time, the program's grantees included top researchers who had been in the field for a long time.

The approach to policy research pioneered by the Substance Abuse Policy Research Program has been replicated in other Robert Wood Johnson Foundation policy research initiatives, notably in childhood obesity prevention and public health law and policy. Specific processes and systems developed by the Substance Abuse Policy Research Program, such as its communications process and internal knowledge management system, have been applied to and adapted by other national programs.

Although the sustainability of substance abuse policy research by other funders remains a question, the contributions of the program's grantees and overarching syntheses and communications efforts made to science, practice, and policy will contribute to improving health and health care for years to come.

Notes

1. See the Substance Abuse Policy Research Program Web site, http://www.the Substance Abuse Policy Research Program.org.
2. DiFranza, J. R., Savageau, J. A., and Fletcher, K. "Enforcement of Underage Laws as a Predictor of Daily Smoking Among Adolescents: A National Study." *BMC Public Health*, 2009, *9*, 107.
3. Ibid.
4. Colorado Senate Bill 95-011.
5. Marine, W. M., and others. *Results of Colorado's Voluntary Alcohol Ignition Interlock Pilot Program (Senate Bill 95-011): Evaluation and Recommendations for Change.* Report to the Colorado General Assembly, May 2000.
6. Merrill, J. O., and others. "Methadone Medical Maintenance in Primary Care: An Implementation Evaluation." *Journal of General Internal Medicine*, 2005, *20*, 344–349.
7. Ibid.
8. Walsh, J. M., Danziger, G., Cangianelli, L. A., and Koehler, D. B. *Driving Under the Influence of Drugs (DUID) Legislation in the United States.* Report for the Robert Wood Johnson Foundation and the American Bar Association Standing Committee on Substance Abuse, November 2002.
9. Walsh, J. M., and Dupont, R. "The Drugged Driving Epidemic." *The Washington Post*, July 17, 2007, p. B8.
10. Lester, B. M., LaGasse, L. L., and Seifer, R. "Cocaine Exposure and Children: The Meaning of Subtle Effects." *Science*, 1998, *282*, 633–634.
11. Larimer, M. E., and others. "Health Care and Public Service Use and Costs Before and After Provision of Housing for Chronically Homeless Persons with Severe Alcohol Problems." *Journal of the American Medical Association*, 2009, *301*, 1349–1357.
12. Ibid.

13. Chaloupka, F. J., and Grossman, M. *Price, Tobacco Control Policies, and Youth Smoking*. National Bureau of Economic Research, Working Paper No. 5740, September 1996.

14. The result was publication of four research agendas: *Policies to Achieve a Smoke-Free Society: A Research Agenda for 2010–2015; Policies to Prevent Alcohol Problems: A Research Agenda for 2010–2015; Policies to Prevent Drug Problems: A Research Agenda for 2010–2015; and Policies for the Treatment of Alcohol and Drug Use Disorders: A Research Agenda for 2010–2015*. All are available at http://www.the Substance Abuse Policy Research Program.org/research_agenda.cfm.

15. Gutman, M. A., Barker, D. C., Samples-Smart, F., and Morley, C. "Evaluation of Active Living Research: Progress and Lessons in Building a New Field." *American Journal of Public Health,* 2009, *36,* S22–S33.

16. The Lewin Group. *Reassessment of the Substance Abuse Policy Research Program*. Unpublished report, 1999.

—ᨠ—The Editors

David C. Colby, PhD, the vice president of research and evaluation at the Robert Wood Johnson Foundation, leads a team dedicated to improving the nation's ability to understand key health and health care issues so that informed decisions can be made concerning the way Americans maintain health and obtain health care. His team also assesses how the Foundation is doing through evaluations, performance measures and score cards, and makes those assessments public. He came to the Foundation in January 1998 after nine years of service with the Medicare Payment Advisory Commission and the Physicians Payment Review Commission, where he was deputy director. Earlier he taught at the University of Maryland Baltimore County, Williams College, and State University College at Buffalo. He was an associate editor of the *Journal of Health Politics, Policy and Law* from 1995 to 2002. He received his doctorate in political science from the University of Illinois, a master of arts from Ohio University, and a bachelor of arts from Ohio Wesleyan University.

Stephen L. Isaacs, JD, is a partner in Isaacs/Jellinek, a San Francisco-based consulting firm, and president of Health Policy Associates, Inc. A former professor of public health at Columbia University and founding director of its Development Law and Policy Program, he has written extensively for professional and popular audiences. His book, *The Consumer's Legal Guide to Today's Health Care*, was reviewed as "the single best guide to the health care system in print today." His articles have been widely syndicated and have appeared in law reviews and health policy journals. He also provides technical assistance internationally on health law, civil society, and social policy. A graduate of Brown University and Columbia Law School, Isaacs served as vice president of International Planned Parenthood's Western Hemisphere Region, practiced health law, and spent four years in Thailand as a program officer for the U.S. Agency for International Development.

—∿—The Contributors

David G. Altman, PhD, is executive vice president of research, innovation, and product development at the Center for Creative Leadership, a global nonprofit organization. Previously, he spent twenty years in academia, ten years as professor (and associate professor) of public health sciences and of pediatrics at the Wake Forest University School of Medicine in Winston-Salem, North Carolina, and ten years as a senior research scientist (and post-doctoral fellow and research associate) at the Stanford University Center for Research in Disease Prevention in Palo Alto, California. Altman received his master's and doctoral degrees in social ecology from the University of California, Irvine, and his bachelor's degree in psychology from the University of California, Santa Barbara. He served fifteen years as national program director of the Robert Wood Johnson Foundation Substance Abuse Policy Research Program. He currently serves as co-director of the national Robert Wood Johnson Foundation Ladder to Leadership program and the Robert Wood Johnson Foundation Executive Nurse Fellows Program. Altman is a fellow of three divisions in the American Psychological Association and of the Society of Behavioral Medicine (SBM). He is also a member of the American Public Health Association, the Council on Epidemiology and Prevention of the American Heart Association, the Society of Public Health Education, and the Academy of Behavioral Medicine Research.

Will Bunch is the senior writer for the *Philadelphia Daily News* and its former political writer, gaining national recognition for his scoops on 9/11 and the war in Iraq. Before coming to

Philadelphia, Bunch was a key member of the *New York Newsday* team that won the 1992 Pulitzer Prize for spot news reporting. His magazine articles have appeared in a number of national and regional publications, including the *New York Times Magazine*. Bunch is also the author of three books, including *The Backlash: Right-Wing Radicals, High-Def Hucksters, and Paranoid Politics in the Age of Obama.*

Digby Diehl is a writer, literary collaborator, and television, print, and Internet journalist. His book credits include *Patti LuPone: A Memoir*, written in collaboration with one of Broadway's foremost leading ladies; *Priceless Memories*, the autobiography of Bob Barker; *Remembering Grace*, a look back at the life of Grace Kelly (with Kay Diehl); the novel *Soapsuds*, written with Finola Hughes; *Angel on My Shoulder*, the autobiography of singer Natalie Cole; *The Million Dollar Mermaid*, the autobiography of MGM star Esther Williams; *Tales from the Crypt*, the history of the popular comic book, movie, and television series; and *A Spy for All Seasons*, the biography of former CIA officer Duane Clarridge. For eleven years, Diehl was the literary correspondent for ABC-TV's Good Morning America, and he was the book editor for the Home Page show on MSNBC. Previously the entertainment editor for KCBS television in Los Angeles, he was a writer for the Emmys and for the soap opera Santa Barbara, book editor of the *Los Angeles Herald-Examiner*, editor-in-chief of art book publisher Harry N. Abrams, and the founding book editor of the *Los Angeles Times Book Review*. Diehl holds a master's degree in theater from UCLA and a bachelor's degree in American studies from Rutgers University, where he was a Henry Rutgers Scholar.

Susan James Frye, MM, is a grants administrator at the Center for Creative Leadership, a global nonprofit enterprise dedicated to advancing the understanding, practice, and development of leadership for the benefit of society worldwide. In her role, she supports the center's grant-seeking work on a three-year, million-dollar, capacity-building grant to expand the center's reach to underserved populations and take its research agenda to a new level. Previously, Frye was grants administrator for the Robert Wood Johnson Foundation's Substance Abuse Policy Research Program (SAPRP), where she partnered with the deputy director in the management of operations of the National Program Office and project-managed and copyedited publications such as SAPRP's substance abuse policy research agendas and Knowledge Assets. Formerly, Frye worked in music education and publishing and wrote early childhood music curricula, fourteen children's books, and articles for teachers and families of young children.

Marjorie A. Gutman, PhD, leads a consulting firm and serves as principal investigator on several evaluation projects through Gutman Research Associates, which specializes in developing and reviewing programs and in designing and conducting evaluations for health philanthropies, government agencies, universities, and community-based organizations, as well as through her affiliation with the Treatment Research Institute at the University of Pennsylvania School of Medicine, where she holds an adjunct faculty position. Gutman's current work is built on twenty-five years of experience in university, philanthropy, and other organizational settings developing, guiding, and evaluating local and national prevention programs with an emphasis on policy and environmental approaches to substance abuse (including tobacco) and childhood obesity, as well as multiservice programs for low-income families through her work at the Treatment Research Institute, the University of Pennsylvania, the Robert Wood Johnson Foundation, the New Jersey State Department of Health, and the State University of New York's Health Sciences Center in Brooklyn. She has served on major commissions, including the Philadelphia Mayor's Blue Ribbon Commission on Child Behavioral Health and the United Way Task Force on Impact. Gutman holds a doctorate in philosophy (applied social psychology) from

New York University and a bachelor's degree from the University of California at Berkeley.

Risa Lavizzo-Mourey, MD, MBA, is the fourth president and chief executive officer of the Robert Wood Johnson Foundation, a position she assumed in January 2003. Under her leadership, the Foundation implemented a defining framework that focuses its mission to improve the health and health care of all Americans and sets bold objectives in nursing, health care disparities, and childhood obesity, as well as improving public health and quality in the health care system. She originally joined the staff in April 2001 as the senior vice president and director of the health care group. Prior to coming to the Foundation, Lavizzo-Mourey was the Sylvan Eisman Professor of Medicine and Health Care Systems at the University of Pennsylvania and director of the Institute on Aging. Lavizzo-Mourey was the deputy administrator of the Agency for Health Care Policy and Research, now known as the Agency for Health Care Research and Quality. Lavizzo-Mourey is the author of numerous articles and several books, has received many awards and honorary doctorates, and frequently appears on national radio and television. A member of the Institute of Medicine of the National Academy of Sciences, she earned her medical degree at Harvard Medical School followed by a master's in business administration at the University of Pennsylvania's Wharton School. After completing a residency in internal medicine at Brigham and Women's Hospital in Boston, Lavizzo-Mourey was a Robert Wood Johnson Clinical Scholar at the University of Pennsylvania, where she also received her geriatrics training.

Carolyn Newbergh is a Northern California writer who has covered health care trends and policy issues for more than twenty years. Her freelance work has appeared in numerous print and online publications. As a reporter for the *Oakland Tribune,* she wrote articles on health care delivery for the poor, emergency room violence, AIDS, and the impact of crack cocaine on the children of addicts. She was also an investigative reporter for the *Tribune*, winning prestigious honors for a series on how consultants intentionally cover up earthquake hazards in California.

Prabhu Ponkshe is president of Health Matrix, Inc., a communications consulting firm that focuses on science, policy, and health care issues. He is a communications consultant for several Robert Wood Johnson Foundation programs, including the Substance Abuse Policy Research Program (SAPRP), the Healthy Eating Research and Active Living Research programs, and the Public Health Law Research program. For all programs, Ponkshe monitors the public and policy debate to provide strategic communications input from funding research through promoting research results. He has previously held senior positions in major health organizations and a health communications firm specializing in government consulting and has been an independent media relations consultant to major national advocacy groups, such as the American Heart Association (AHA), the Coalition on Smoking OR Health, and the American Red Cross. Ponkshe was also director of public relations at the AHA's National Center. He started his career as a reporter for Reuters. He has a master's degree in mass communications and a degree in law.

Sara Solovitch is a writer whose stories have appeared in *Esquire*, *Wired*, *Outside*, and other publications. She has been a staff reporter at several major newspapers, including the *Philadelphia Inquirer*, and has had numerous stories published in the *Washington Post* and the *Los Angeles Times*. For six years, she wrote a weekly column on children's health for the *San Jose Mercury-News*. Solovitch has taught writing and journalism at all levels from elementary school to the graduate program in science communication at the University of California, Santa Cruz. She is currently an editor at *Bay Area Parent*. Her magazine articles have won national awards from the American Society of Journalists and Authors, the National Education Association, and Genetic Alliance. She lives in Santa Cruz, California.

Andrea Williams currently serves as a research associate at the Center for Creative Leadership (CCL). In April 2010 she became deputy director of the Robert Wood Johnson Foundation's Executive Nurse Fellows Program. During her tenure at CCL, she served for fifteen years as deputy director of the Robert Wood Johnson Foundation-funded Substance Abuse Policy Research Program (SAPSP). Prior to joining CCL in 2004, Williams worked for ten years as a research associate at the Wake Forest University School of Medicine (WFUSM) and was involved in multisite evaluations of government-funded public health programs. She holds a bachelor's degree in economics and a master's degree in counseling, both from Wake Forest University.

Irene M. Wielawski is an independent writer and editor specializing in health care and policy topics. She has written extensively on socioeconomic issues in American medicine, particularly the difficulties faced by people without timely access to medical services because of financial, geographic, cultural, and other barriers. Wielawski was a staff writer for nearly twenty years for daily newspapers, most recently, the *Los Angeles Times*, where she was a member of the investigations team. Subsequently, with a research grant from the Robert Wood Johnson Foundation, she tracked local efforts to care for the medically uninsured. Other commissioned projects include producing pediatric medicine segments for public television and an analysis of the Massachusetts health reform law. Her independent work appears in the *New York Times, Los Angeles Times*, and *Kaiser Health News* among daily outlets, on Web sites, and in peer-reviewed journals and books. Wielawski has been a finalist for the Pulitzer Prize for medical reporting and shared in two Los Angeles Times staff Pulitzers, among other honors. She is a founder and current board member of the Association of Health Care Journalists, a reviewer for *Health Affairs*, an outside editor for the *American Journal of Nursing*, and a graduate of Vassar College.

—ᴡ—Index

─୶─Anthology Chapters by Topic 1997 Through Volume XIV

Health Insurance Coverage, Access, and Cost

Overview Chapters

The Politics of Health Care Reform, *Vol. XII* (2009)

Research on Health Insurance Coverage, *Vol. XII* (2009)

Health Services Research, *Vol. XI* (2008)

Efforts to Cover the Uninsured, *Vol. IX* (2006)

Safety-Net Programs, *Vol. IX* (2006)

Cost Containment, *Vol. VII* (2004)

Managed Care, *2001*

Workers' Compensation, *2001*

Emergency Medical Services, *2000*

Academic Medical Centers, *1998–1999*

Medical Malpractice, *1997*

Data Collection/Analysis

Health Tracking, *Vol. VI* (2003)

National Access-to-Care Surveys, *1997*

State and Local Levels/Increasing Enrollment

Enrolling Eligible People in Medicaid and SCHIP, *Vol. XII* (2009)

Health Insurance and Small Business: The Communities in Charge Program, *Vol. IX* (2007)

Medicaid Managed Care, *Vol. IX* (2006)

The Covering Kids Communication Campaign, *Vol. VI* (2003)

Health Insurance for Children, *2000*

Improving State Government Capacity in Health Reform, *1997*

Rural Areas

Dental Health Aides and Therapists in Alaska, *Vol. XIV* (2011)

Improving Health Care in Rural America, *Vol. XII* (2009)

The Southern Rural Access Program, *Vol. IX* (2007)

Primary Care in Rural Areas: The Practice Sights Program, *Vol. VI* (2003)

The Swing Bed Program, *Vol. VI* (2003)

Encouraging Physician Volunteerism: The Reach Out Program, *1997*

Access to Specific Services

Community-Based Dental Education: The Pipeline, Profession, and Practice Program, *Vol. XII* (2009)

Asthma, *Vol. XII* (2009)

AIDS, *Vol. V* (2002)

Tuberculosis Care, *Vol. V* (2002)

Dental Care, *2001*

Mental Health: The Chronic Mental Illness Program, *2000*

Mental Health Services for Youth, *1998–1999*

Health Policy/Public Policy

Shaping Public Policy as a Foundation Approach, *Vol. XII* (2009)

The National Health Policy Forum, *Vol. VII* (2004)

End of Life

The Foundation's End-of-Life Programs, *Vol. VI* (2003)

SUPPORT, *1997*

Public Health

The Turning Point Program, *Vol. VIII* (2005)

Responding to Emergencies: 9/11, Bioterrorism, and Natural Disasters, *Vol. VII* (2004)

Substance Abuse/Addiction Prevention and Treatment

Substance Abuse Policy Research

The Substance Abuse Policy Research Program, *Vol. XIV* (2011)

Tobacco

Smoking Cessation and Pregnant Women (The Smoke-Free Families Program), *Vol. XI* (2008)

The Foundation's Tobacco-Control Strategy and Initiatives, *Vol. VIII* (2005)

The SmokeLess States Program, *Vol. VIII* (2005)

The National Center for Tobacco-Free Kids, *Vol. VI* (2003)

Tobacco Cessation, *Vol. VI* (2003)

The Sundance Conference and Its Aftermath, *2000*

Tobacco Policy Research, *1998–1999*

The National Spit Tobacco Program, *1998–1999*

Drugs and Alcohol

The Foundation's Efforts to Combat Drug Addiction, *Vol. XIII* (2010)

The College Alcohol Study, *Vol. XIII* (2010)

The Evolution of the Foundation's Efforts to Prevent and Treat Addictions, *Vol. IX* (2006)

Working with Head Start (The Free to Grow to Grow Program), *Vol. IX* (2006)

Reducing Underage Drinking, *Vol. VIII* (2005)

Specific Populations

Homeless People

The Health Care for the Homeless Program, *Vol. IX* (2006)

The Homeless Prenatal Program, *Vol. VII* (2004)

The Homeless Families Program, *1997*

Minorities

The United Teen Equity Center, *Vol. XIV* (2011)

Overcoming Language Barriers to Care (*Hablamos Juntos*), *Vol. XIII* (2010)

Increasing Minorities in the Health Professions, *Vol. VII* (2004)

The Minority Medical Education Program, *2000*

Native Americans

The Catholic Social Services Outreach Project in Lakota Sioux Reservations, *Vol. XII* (2009)

Fighting Back and Healthy Nations in Gallup, New Mexico, *Vol. VI* (2003)

Programs to Improve the Health of Native Americans, *Vol. V* (2002)

People in the Criminal Justice System

Young People with Addictions in the Juvenile Justice System (Reclaiming Futures), *Vol. XIII* (2010)

Former Prisoners Reentering Society (Health Link), *Vol. XII* (2009)

Children and Adolescents

Playworks/Sports4Kids, *Vol. XIV* (2011)

Reducing Teenage Pregnancy, *Vol. XI* (2008)

Mentoring Young People, *Vol. XI* (2008)

The Urban Health Initiative, *Vol. XI* (2008)

Students Run L.A., *Vol. IX* (2006)

The National Health Care Purchasing Institute: A Case Study, *Vol. XIII* (2010)

The Role of Failure in Philanthropic Learning, *Vol. XIII* (2010)

Inside the Robert Wood Johnson Foundation

Engaging Coalitions as a Foundation Strategy, *Vol. IX* (2007)

A Ten-Year Retrospective: 1996–2006, *Vol. IX* (2007)

The Foundation: 1974–2002, *Vol. IX* (2007)

National Programs as an Approach to Grantmaking, *Vol. VIII* (2005)

The Foundation's Early Years, *Vol. VII* (2004)

An Interview with Steve Schroeder, *Vol. VI* (2003)

Program-Related Investments, *Vol. V* (2002)

Grantmaking in New Jersey, *Vol. V.* (2002)

Expanding the Focus: Health as an Equal Partner to Health Care, *2001*

Research as a Foundation Strategy, *2000*

Adopting the Substance Abuse Goal, *1998–1999*

Communications

Communications Strategy at the Robert Wood Johnson Foundation, *Vol. XII* (2009)

Communications and the Changing State of Philanthropy, *Vol. IX* (2006)

Getting the Word Out: A Foundation Memoir and Personal Journey by Frank Karel, *2001*

Sound Partners for Community Health, *2001*

The Foundation's Radio and Television Grants, *1998–1999*

The Media and Health Tracking, *1997*

Relations Among Foundations

Partnership Among Foundations, *2001*

The Local Initiative Funding Partners Program, *2000*

Other